ORTHOPEDIC CLINICS OF NORTH AMERICA

www.orthopedic.theclinics.com

Minimally Invasive Surgery

July 2020 • Volume 51 • Number 3

ELSEVIER

1600 John F. Kennedy Boulevard • Suite 1800 • Philadelphia, Pennsylvania, 19103-2899.

http://www.orthopedic.theclinics.com

ORTHOPEDIC CLINICS OF NORTH AMERICA Volume 51, Number 3
July 2020 ISSN 0030-5898, ISBN-13: 978-0-323-79190-8

Editor: Lauren Boyle

Developmental Editor: Kristen Helm

Orthopedic Clinics of North America (ISSN 0030-5898) is published quarterly by Elsevier Inc., 360 Park Avenue South, New York, NY 10010-1710. Months of issue are January, April, July, and October. Business and Editorial Offices: 1600 John F. Kennedy Blvd., Suite 1800, Philadelphia, PA 19103-2899. Customer Service Office: 3251 Riverport Lane, Maryland Heights, MO 63043. Periodicals postage paid at New York, NY and additional mailing offices. Subscription prices are $344.00 per year for (US individuals), $786.00 per year for (US institutions), $403.00 per year (Canadian individuals), $960.00 per year (Canadian institutions), $471.00 per year (international individuals), $960.00 per year (international institutions), $100.00 per year (US students), $100.00 per year for (Canadian students), $220.00 per year for (international students). Foreign air speed delivery is included in all *Clinics* subscription prices. All prices are subject to change without notice. **POSTMASTER:** Send change of address to *Orthopedic Clinics of North America*, **Elsevier Health Sciences Division, Subscription Customer Service, 3251 Riverport Lane, Maryland Heights, MO 63043. Customer Service (orders, claims, online, change of address): Elsevier Health Sciences Division, Subscription Customer Service, 3251 Riverport Lane, Maryland Heights, MO 63043. Tel: 1-800-654-2452 (U.S. and Canada); 314-447-8871 (outside U.S. and Canada). Fax: 314-447-8029. E-mail:** journalscustomerservice-usa@elsevier.com **(for print support);** journalsonlinesupport-usa@elsevier.com **(for online support).**

Reprints. For copies of 100 or more, of articles in this publication, please contact the Commercial Reprints Department, Elsevier Inc., 360 Park Avenue South, New York, NY 10010-1710. Tel.: 212-633-3874; Fax: 212-633-3820; E-mail: reprints@elsevier.com.

Orthopedic Clinics of North America is covered in *MEDLINE/PubMed* (*Index Medicus*), *Cinahl, Excerpta Medica,* and *Cumulative Index to Nursing and Allied Health Literature.*

EDITORIAL BOARD

CONTRIBUTORS

AUTHORS

RYAN S. BAILEY, MD
Resident Physician, Department of
Orthopaedic Surgery, Saint Louis University,
St Louis, Missouri, USA

KATHERINE BARTUSH, MD
Steadman Philippon Research Institute, Vail,
Colorado, USA

LOUISE REID BOYCE NICHOLS, MD,
FAAOS
Pediatric Orthopaedic Surgeon, Department
of Orthopaedic Surgery, Nemours Al duPont
Hospital for Children, Wilmington, Delaware,
USA

JAMES CALANDRUCCIO, MD
Associate Professor, Department of
Orthopaedic Surgery and Biomedical
Engineering, University of Tennessee-
Campbell Clinic, Memphis, Tennessee, USA

JAMES CHAMBERS, MD
PGY-4 Orthopaedic Resident, Department of
Orthopaedic Surgery and Biomedical
Engineering, University of Tennessee-
Campbell Clinic, Memphis, Tennessee, USA

THOMAS CLANTON, MD
Medical Director, Foot and Ankle Sports
Medicine, The Steadman Clinic and Steadman
Philippon Research Institute, Vail, Colorado,
USA

JONATHAN DAY, MS
Hospital for Special Surgery, New York,
New York, USA

RAYMOND J. GARDOCKI, MD
Assistant Professor, Department of
Orthopaedic Surgery and Biomedical
Engineering, University of Tennessee-
Campbell Clinic, Memphis, Tennessee, USA

CHARLES L. GETZ, MD
Associate Professor, Shoulder and Elbow
Division, Rothman Orthopaedic Institute,
Philadelphia, Pennsylvania, USA

ISHVINDER S. GREWAL, FRCS
Parkland Memorial Hospital, University of
Texas Southwestern, Dallas, Texas, USA

MARISSA D. JAMIESON, MD
Steadman Philippon Research Institute, Vail,
Colorado, USA

BAO-QUYNH JILLIAN, MD
Division of Plastic and Reconstructive Surgery,
Department of Surgery, UT Health San
Antonio, San Antonio, Texas, USA

ANNE HOLLY JOHNSON, MD
Hospital for Special Surgery, New York, New
York, USA

CHRISTOPHER D. JOYCE, MD
Shoulder and Elbow Fellow, Rothman
Orthopaedic Institute, Philadelphia,
Pennsylvania, USA

EFSTATHIOS KARAMANOS, MD
Division of Plastic and Reconstructive Surgery,
Department of Surgery, UT Health San
Antonio, San Antonio, Texas, USA

YOUNG W. KWON, MD, PhD
Department of Orthopaedic Surgery, NYU
Grossman School of Medicine, NYU Langone
Orthopedic Hospital, New York, New York,
USA

JOHN LAWRENCE MARSH, MD
Department Head, Professor, Carroll B Larson
Chair, Department of Orthopedics and
Rehabilitation, University of Iowa Hospitals
and Clinics, University of Iowa, Iowa City,
Iowa, USA

JASON P. MORA, DO
Fellow, Adult Reconstruction, Department of
Orthopedic Surgery, Lenox Hill Hospital,
Northwell Health, New York, New York, USA

NICKOLAS NAHM, MD
Fellow, International Center for Limb
Lengthening, Rubin Institute for Advanced
Orthopaedics, Sinai Hospital of Baltimore,
Baltimore, Maryland, USA

CATHERINE R. OLINGER, MD
PGY-5 Resident, Department of Orthopaedic
Surgery and Biomedical Engineering,
University of Tennessee-Campbell Clinic,
Memphis, Tennessee, USA

TAYLOR PATE, MD
Radiology Resident, Department of
Orthopaedic Surgery and Biomedical
Engineering, University of Tennessee-
Campbell Clinic, Memphis, Tennessee, USA

DAVID PERSON, MD
The Hand Center of San Antonio, San
Antonio, Texas, USA

AKI PURYEAR, MD
Associate Professor, Department of
Orthopaedic Surgery, Saint Louis University,
St Louis, Missouri, USA

GABRIELLE S. RAY, BA
Tufts University School of Medicine, Boston,
Massachusetts, USA

YOAV ROSENTHAL, MD
Department of Orthopaedic
Surgery, Affiliated with Tel Aviv
University, Rabin Medical Center, Petah
Tikva, Israel

OLIVER N. SCHIPPER, MD
Anderson Orthopaedic Clinic, Arlington,
Virginia, USA

GILES R. SCUDERI, MD, FAAOS, FACS
Fellowship Director, Adult Reconstruction,
Department of Orthopedic Surgery, Lenox Hill
Hospital, Northwell, Northwell Health
Orthopaedic Institute at MEETH, New York,
New York, USA

INGRID K. STAKE, MD
Department of Orthopaedic Surgery, Ostfold
Hospital Trust, Norway and Steadman
Philippon Research Institute, Vail, Colorado,
USA

ADAM J. STARR, MD
Parkland Memorial Hospital, University
of Texas Southwestern, Dallas, Texas,
USA

BRANDON G. WILKINSON, MD
Resident Physician, Department of
Orthopedics and Rehabilitation, University of
Iowa Hospitals and Clinics, University of Iowa,
Iowa City, Iowa, USA

CONTENTS

Knee and Hip Reconstruction
Patrick C. Toy and William M. Mihalko

A surgical approach to total knee arthroplasty has been at the forefront of
many conversations. Surgeons used the medial parapatellar approach for its familiarity of anatomy, reliability, and ability to convert to a more extensile
approach. This article reviews the current literature and information regarding
the effect of surgical approach on patients' outcomes. The results of the limited
medial parapatellar, subvastus, midvastus, and quadriceps-sparing approaches
were analyzed. All techniques can provide adequate exposure with successful
outcomes. It is recommended that a surgeon perform the approach with which
they are most comfortable, because that will likely yield the best patient
outcome.

Trauma
John C. Weinlein and Michael J. Beebe

Percutaneous reduction and fixation of pelvic ring fractures is now widely
accepted as a safe and effective treatment method. The only exception remains reduction and fixation of pubic symphyseal injuries. Several units from
China and one from Spain have published clinical and biomechanical studies
supporting percutaneous reduction and fixation of the pubic symphysis with
various screw configurations. The initial clinical results are promising. Biomechanical data show there is little difference between plate and screw fixation.
We review the current literature and also present a case performed by our-
selves using this novel technique.

Minimally invasive surgical techniques are increasingly used for definitive treatment of displaced intra-articular calcaneal fractures. These approaches have
been shown to minimize soft tissue injury, preserve blood supply, and decrease
operative time. These methods can be applied to all calcaneal fractures and
have particular advantages in patients with higher than usual risks to the soft
tissues. The literature suggests that results of limited soft tissue dissection approaches provide equivalent outcomes to those obtained with the extensile
lateral approach. We predict that as imaging and other techniques continue
to improve, more calcaneal fractures will be treated by these appealing safer
techniques.

Arthroscopic Latarjet is a relatively new, but viable option for the treatment of anterior shoulder instability. Arthroscopic Latarjet has the advantage of faster recovery, reduced stiffness, identification of additional shoulder pathology, and improved cosmesis when compared with open Latarjet. By the majority of clinical and radiographic parameters, arthroscopic Latarjet produces equivalent outcomes compared with open Latarjet. A relatively substantial learning curve for arthroscopic Latarjet exists at about 25 cases; however, multiple studies have demonstrated comparable outcomes and surgical time after the learning curve.

Traditionally, total shoulder arthroplasty is performed through the deltopectoral approach with violation of the subscapularis tendon. In order to reduce the incidence of postoperative subscapularis dysfunction, the subscapularis-sparing approach, performed entirely through the rotator interval, was developed. This technique allows earlier rehabilitation and may potentially prevent subsequent subscapularis insufficiency and clinical failures.

Achilles tendon rupture is an increasingly common problem with an aging population participating in high-level physical activities. Appropriate treatment has been debated for decades, but good outcomes have been reported after conservative and surgical management. The development of minimally invasive surgical techniques for Achilles repair has reduced the incidence of complications and maintained the high level of function reported after open surgery. The Achilles Midsubstance SpeedBridge repair is a newer minimally invasive technique that has demonstrated promising results and is the authors' preferred treatment of Achilles tendon rupture in athletes and active patients.

This article presents the indications, contraindications, preoperative surgical planning, surgical technique, and postoperative management of some of the most common percutaneous procedures in orthopedic foot and ankle surgery. The background of each procedure also is presented, supported by the latest in published literature to educate surgeons. Such topics include percutaneous bunionectomy, lesser toe deformity and bunionette correction, calcaneal osteotomy, cheilectomy, and first metatarsophalangeal joint arthrodesis.

When the guidelines of the North American Spine Society concerning deep venous thrombosis (DVT) prophylaxis were followed, only 2 (0.63%) of 315 patients with minimally invasive transforaminal lumbar interbody fusions developed DVT complications over a 9-year period. Based on these findings, mechanical DVT prophylaxis appears to be adequate in patients undergoing elective spinal surgery, with no current support for pharmacologic prophylaxis.

MINIMALLY INVASIVE SURGERY

PREFACE

Minimally Invasive Surgery: Is Less More?

Over the past few decades, minimally invasive surgery has become increasingly common across all medical specialties, and orthopedics is no exception. New research and technologies have led to improved methods of joint replacement, treatment of traumatic injuries, arthroscopic treatment of sports injuries, and endoscopic or arthroscopic treatment of complex musculoskeletal conditions, such as congenital anomalies and neurosurgical-associated conditions. The authors of this issue have provided valuable information about procedures ranging from endoscopic carpal tunnel release to minimally invasive total joint arthroplasty.

Between 2012 and 2015, there was a 47% increase in elective outpatient total joint arthroplasty, and it is expected that there will be a 77% growth over the next 10 years. Mora and Scuderi provide a review of the most current literature and information regarding the effect of the surgical approach (limited medial parapatellar, subvastus, midvastus, and quadriceps-sparing) on the outcomes of total knee arthroplasty.

Minimally invasive surgical techniques are being increasingly used for definitive treatment of traumatic injuries, including fractures. Grewal and Starr, and Wilkinson and Marsh have given descriptions of minimally invasive techniques for fixation of fractures of the pelvis and calcaneus, respectively.

Minimally invasive techniques are especially beneficial for skeletally immature patients. In addition to speeding recovery and decreasing morbidity, these techniques can help preserve blood supply and physeal function. Pediatric spine injuries often result from high-energy mechanisms and are associated with other serious injuries. Bailey and Puryear discuss percutaneous pedicle screw instrumentation, temporary fixation without fusion, and its expanding role in the treatment of pediatric spine fractures. Lower-extremity deformities in children rely on osteotomies for correction, and Nahm and Nichols identify the advantages and indications for percutaneous osteotomies, such as drill-hole osteotomy,

corticotomy, and Gigli-saw osteotomies. They also emphasize the technically demanding nature of these techniques and the need for an experienced surgeon for their use.

A variety of minimally invasive techniques are used in hand surgery, and most hand procedures are done as outpatient procedures, including wide-awake in-office endoscopic carpal tunnel release. Karamanos and Person describe the technical considerations for the single incision, antegrade approach to endoscopic carpal tunnel release using the SEGWay system and technique, while Chambers, Pate, and Calandruccio report the outcomes and complications of office-based percutaneous for Dupuytren contracture release.

Although arthroscopic shoulder surgery has been slower to develop than that of the knee or hip, Getz and Joyce report that the arthroscopic Latarjet procedure has the advantage of faster recovery, reduced stiffness, identification of additional shoulder pathology, and improved cosmesis when compared with open Latarjet procedures. They estimated a learning curve of about 25 cases. Just as arthroscopic shoulder procedures have lagged behind those of the knee and hip, minimally invasive total shoulder arthroplasty is relatively new. Rosenthal and Kwon discuss the development of the subscapularis-sparing approach, performed entirely through the rotator interval to reduce the frequency of postoperative subscapularis dysfunction and clinical failures.

Achilles tendon injuries are common in athletes and are becoming more frequent in an aging population. Good outcomes have been reported after both conservative and surgical management, but the development of minimally invasive surgical techniques for Achilles repair has reduced the frequency of complications and maintained the high level of function reported after open surgery. Clanton and colleagues describe their technique and report outcomes with the Achilles Midsubstance SpeedBridge repair. A number of other minimally invasive procedures are used in foot

Orthop Clin N Am 51 (2020) xiii–xiv
https://doi.org/10.1016/j.ocl.2020.04.001
0030-5898/20/© 2020 Published by Elsevier Inc.

and ankle surgery. Schipper and colleagues present the indications, contraindications, preoperative surgical planning, surgical technique, and postoperative management of some of the most common percutaneous procedures (percutaneous bunionectomy, lesser toe deformity and bunionette correction, calcaneal osteotomy, cheilectomy, and first metatarsophalangeal joint arthrodesis). They also provide the background of each procedure supported by the latest in published literature.

Finally, in a special article, Olinger and Gardocki give information on the development of deep venous thrombosis (DVT) and pulmonary embolism after minimally invasive transforaminal lumbar interbody fusion. Of 315 patients, only two (<1%) developed DVT complications over a 9-year period. These results led the authors to conclude that mechanical DVT prophylaxis appears to be adequate in patients undergoing elective spinal surgery, with no current support for pharmacologic prophylaxis.

Overall, this collection of articles brings to light the usefulness of minimally invasive orthopedic procedures and provides information concerning indications, techniques, outcomes, and complications. We hope this information will be helpful to you to improve outcomes and decrease complications in your patients.

Frederick M. Azar, MD
Department of Orthopaedic Surgery &
Biomedical Engineering
University of Tennessee–
Campbell Clinic
1211 Union Avenue, Suite 510
Memphis, TN 38104, USA

E-mail address:
fazar@campbellclinic.com

Knee and Hip Reconstruction

Minimally Invasive Total Knee Arthroplasty
Does Surgical Technique Actually Impact the Outcome?

Jason P. Mora, DO[a], Giles R. Scuderi, MD[b],*

KEYWORDS

- Minimally invasive surgery • Total knee arthroplasty • Medial parapatellar • Quad sparing
- Mini medial parapatellar • Midvastus • Subvastus • Outcomes

KEY POINTS

- There are various minimally invasive surgical approaches for performing a total knee arthroplasty, including the limited medial parapatellar, subvastus, midvastus, and quadriceps-sparing approaches.
- When comparing the conventional medial parapatellar approach with minimally invasive techniques, there may be a benefit to range of motion and Knee Society scores in the early postoperative period.
- The benefits quickly even out and there seem to be no significant difference in outcomes between the approaches in the late postoperative period.
- All approaches are proven to be successful; our recommendation is for a surgeon to perform the approach with which they are most comfortable, because that should yield the best patient outcome.

INTRODUCTION

Currently, the topic of surgical approach for total knee arthroplasty (TKA) has been at the forefront of many conversations. Traditionally, surgeons used the medial parapatellar approach for its familiarity of anatomy, reliability, and ability to easily convert to a more extensile approach. Over the years, surgeons have tried to modify or improve surgical approaches to positively impact both intraoperative outcomes and postoperative function. In the early 1990s, surgeons began developing minimally invasive surgical (MIS) techniques to improve patient outcomes by minimizing dissection to potentially decrease the amount of soft tissue disruption and decrease blood loss, thus decreasing a patient's time to postoperative recovery of function.[1] Historically, these techniques were developed for the performance of unicompartmental knee arthroplasty. Repicci and colleagues[1] were able to popularize the minimally invasive approach after favorable early results from their series of unicompartmental knee arthroplasties performed through a 10-cm skin incision and limited medial capsular arthrotomy.

Recently, there has been interest in analyzing the validity of the hypothetical improvements in outcome and function with less invasive surgery. Numerous studies have examined the various commonly used surgical approaches and evaluated their effect on clinical outcomes. The

[a] Adult Reconstruction, Department of Orthopedic Surgery, Lenox Hill Hospital, Northwell, Northwell Health Orthopaedic Institute at MEETH, 210 East 64th Street, 4th Floor, New York, NY 10065, USA; [b] Adult Reconstruction, Department of Orthopedic Surgery, Lenox Hill Hospital, Northwell, 130 East 77th Street, 11th Floor, New York, NY 10075, USA
* Corresponding author.
E-mail address: gscuderi@northwell.edu

Orthop Clin N Am 51 (2020) 303–315
https://doi.org/10.1016/j.ocl.2020.02.009

long-term benefits of each MIS approach have been scrutinized to compare the accuracy of implant placement, fixation, postoperative complication, and ultimately functional outcome.

The current medical climate relies heavily on bundle payments, cost effectiveness, and patient outcomes, and, as a result, surgeons must evaluate all aspects of patient care. Moreover, some patients are increasingly inquiring about a surgeon's ability and willingness to perform a TKA through a particular surgical approach using advanced technologies. Therefore, it is important for surgeons to be able to thoroughly discuss with patients the benefits and pitfalls to all surgical approaches as they pertain to a patient's recovery and ultimate outcome. The purpose of this article is to review the most current literature available and compare how surgical approaches, whether it is traditional or minimally invasive techniques, impact postoperative outcomes.

TRADITIONAL APPROACH
Medial Parapatellar Arthrotomy
The traditional medial parapatellar arthrotomy has been the workhorse for TKA for many decades. Since its beginning, when it was originally described by von Langenbeck to its modifications by Sir Robert Jones and John Insall, it has proven to be a reliable approach.[2] It provides adequate visualization for implantation of a total knee prosthesis with appropriate alignment, size, and balance.

This approach gains access into the knee joint by making an incision approximately 8 to 10 cm proximal to the superior pole of the patella. The incision incorporates a small sleeve of the medial quadriceps tendon to displace the vastus medialis medially and extensor mechanism with the patella laterally. As the quadriceps tendon incision is brought distally to the patella, there are some variations to the approach. Although some surgeons prefer to come around the medial border of the patella with a curvilinear incision, Insall preferred a vertical incision directly over the medial border of the patella and subperiosteally dissecting the medial capsule from the medial border of the patella. The medial arthrotomy is then continued distally along the medial edge of the patella tendon adjacent to the tibial tubercle.[3]

Once the arthrotomy is made, visualization of the suprapatellar pouch and infrapatellar fat pad is achieved. With retraction, knee flexion, and lateral subluxation of the patella, the knee joint is exposed. With a stiff knee and limited exposure, the medial parapatellar arthrotomy can easily be extended or incorporated into more extensile approaches (Fig. 1).

MINIMALLY INVASIVE APPROACHES
Quadriceps-Sparing Approach
In the early 2000s, the quadriceps-sparing approach was developed. The impetus of its development was to create a true anatomic approach without violation of the extensor mechanism. This approach begins with a 10-cm anterior skin incision. Then, a mini parapatellar capsular incision is made starting at the superior pole of the patella and continuing to 2 cm distal to the tibial joint line.[4] The differentiating factor of this approach is that it does not violate any fibers of the quadriceps muscle. This approach was initially popular in performing unicompartmental knee arthroplasty with the use of minimally invasive instruments.[5] The quadriceps-sparing approach was later adopted by some surgeons to perform TKA. Without having to further disrupt soft tissue planes, patients may have an easier recovery and decreased blood loss plus increased range of motion (ROM).[1]

To perform this technique, companies began developing smaller specialized surgical instruments, including retractors, alignment guides, and cutting blocks, to perform the surgery within a smaller operative field with the same accuracy in bone preparation and implant position as with a conventional approach.[6] Early on, surgeons

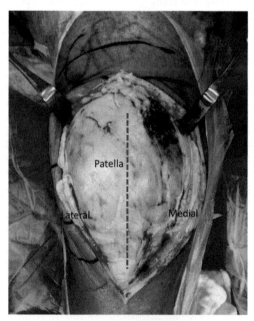

Fig. 1. Traditional medial parapatellar arthrotomy. *Red dashed line* signifies incision.

quickly appreciated the learning curve for this technique as many failures were being discovered, which seemed to be attributable to technical errors.[1] However, through repetition and advances in instrumentation, some surgeons have adopted this technique in very select patients. Patient selection and surgeon experience play an important role when choosing this approach. Iatrogenic complications such as collateral ligament rupture, cement retention, and patella tendon avulsions all decrease with advanced surgical experience (**Fig. 2**).[7]

Mini Subvastus Approach

Historically, the subvastus approach has been recognized as a reasonable approach for most primary TKA. This approach was typically done through an anterior midline skin incision. Modifications have been made to gain the necessary exposure without extensive skin incisions.[8] However, owing to the maintained integrity of the proximal medial muscular sleeve, many surgeons have abandoned this approach for revision reconstructive procedures because of its limited extensile exposure.[1]

The approach uses a straight anterior midline skin incision. The subcutaneous dissection is carried out down to the retinacular capsular layer, exposing the extensor mechanism. The difference from the traditional medial parapatellar approach lies within its deep incision. The deep subcutaneous layer is developed as a medial

flap at the lower border of the vastus medialis muscle (VMO). The VMO has an insertion that is found at a 50° angle to the midbody of the patella.[9] The arthrotomy begins along the medial border of the patella tendon from its insertion at the tibial tubercle and extends proximally to the insertion of the VMO at the medial patella border. The incision is then continued in a medial direction along the lower border of the muscular belly of the VMO. The VMO and patella tendon are retracted laterally and as the knee is brought to 90° of flexion the patella is subluxed laterally, exposing the knee joint. To facilitate exposure the suprapatella plica is incised (**Fig. 3**).

Mini Midvastus Approach

With the extensile limitations that are inherent to the subvastus approach and the difficulty of the quadriceps-sparing approach, some surgeons have used a midvastus approach for its potential ease.[10] This approach has been seen as a fine middle ground between the medial parapatellar and the subvastus approaches for primary TKA.[11] An anterior midline skin incision provides exposure to the extensor mechanism with subcutaneous dissection. The arthrotomy begins along the medial border of the patella tendon from its insertion at the tibial tubercle and extends proximally to the insertion of the VMO at the medial patella border. Visualization of the superior medial border of the patella is

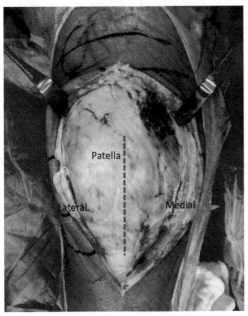

Fig. 2. Quadriceps-sparing arthrotomy. *Red dashed line* signifies incision.

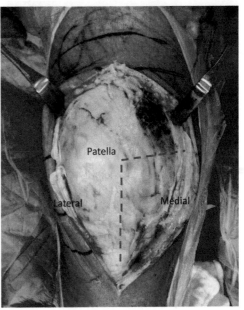

Fig. 3. Mini subvastus arthrotomy. Red dashed line signifies incision.

paramount, because you must find the insertion fibers of the VMO.[1] An incision is made parallel with the fibers of the VMO directed from the superior medial border of the patella into and along the muscle fibers. As the knee is brought into flexion and the patella subluxed laterally, the knee joint is exposed as the fibers of the VMO split. The degree of proximal muscle split provides exposure to the knee joint (Fig. 4).

Limited Medial Parapatellar Arthrotomy

The limited medial parapatellar arthrotomy has evolved from the traditional arthrotomy by limiting the amount of dissection or incision into the quadriceps tendon. This procedure relies on the same soft tissue landmarks and tissue planes as the traditional approach. The limited parapatellar arthrotomy takes advantage of the anatomy with selective position of retractors and allows creation of a mobile window to gain access into the knee joint.[1] The purpose of the limited approach is to minimize the skin incision and minimize the length of the arthrotomy to only what is required for visualization and appropriate placement of the implants.

An anterior midline incision is made; however, the incision spans from just proximal to the superior pole of the patella and continues distantly to the tibial tubercle. Subcutaneous dissection exposes the capsular retinacular layer. A medial parapatellar arthrotomy is created beginning 2 to 4 cm proximal to the superior pole of the

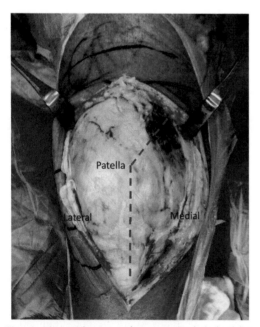

Fig. 4. Mini midvastus arthrotomy. *Red dashed line* signifies incision.

patella, leaving a small sleeve of quadriceps tendon attached to the VMO.[1] The arthrotomy is continued along the medial border of the patella and patella tendon continuing down the tibial tubercle.

To further facilitate exposed if needed, the incision of both skin and arthrotomy can be easily extended to gain adequate exposure. The learning curve for this approach was quantified by King and colleagues[1] and found to be approximately 50 TKA performed by high-volume surgeons. However, owing to the ability to easily extend the incision, this procedure has proved to be a friendly approach for surgeons.

CLINICAL OUTCOMES
Early Versus Late Recovery

After reviewing the most recent literature and gathering the clinical outcomes, the reports remain consistent (Table 1). A systematic review by Bourke and colleagues[12] showed no difference in clinical outcomes when comparing the medial parapatellar and subvastus approaches. These findings were similar to the quadriceps-sparing techniques as well. No difference was found with respect to early recovery when comparing quad-sparing and mini subvastus approach.[13]

Yao and colleagues[14] reported on the ability to regain quadriceps strength when comparing the mini subvastus and traditional medial parapatellar approaches. They found that patients treated with the mini subvastus approach were able to perform a straight leg raise faster than the control group. However, strength recovery was not exponential and quickly plateaued after 2 weeks postoperatively.

Some studies have attempted to discover benefits when comparing different MIS techniques. Bonutti and colleagues[8] reported on a prospective, randomized, controlled trial of bilateral TKA with one side having a midvastus and the other having a subvastus. There was no difference observed between the 2 approaches. Cho and colleagues[15] reported on a comparison of a mini midvastus group with a mini medial parapatellar and found that quadriceps force was stronger in the mini midvastus group when compared with the limited medial parapatellar group at 6 weeks. Interestingly, the more limited medial parapatellar group had greater quadriceps recovery than the mini midvastus group during the first 6 weeks to 3 months. This difference was not evident over time; at 1 year postoperatively, both groups had no significant differences in quadriceps strength.

Table 1
Summary of clinical outcomes

Early vs Late Recovery	ROM	KS Scores	Length of Incision and Cosmesis	Duration of Surgery
Bourke et al showed no difference comparing medial parapatellar and subvastus approach	Obaid-ur-Rahman and Amin found greater ROM in a quadriceps-sparing approach.	Obaid-ur-Rahman and Amin reported higher KS scores in the quadriceps-sparing group when compared with the conventional approach at 1 mo and 3 mo but no differences after 3 mo.	Smith et al demonstrated a significantly smaller length of the skin incision in the MIS groups (10–13 cm in the MIS groups and >13 cm in the conventional group).	Peng et al in a meta-analysis reported an increase in the duration of surgery (>18 minutes for MIS).
Yao et al found the mini subvastus group was able to perform an SLR faster than the control group in <2 wk postoperatively	Yao et al also found early ROM improvements in their MIS group. At 1 and 3 d, the mini subvastus group had improved ROM, but this difference normalized by 14 d.	Peng et al showed improvements in KS scores for the quadriceps-sparing group compared with the conventional group at 3 mo and 2 y. No subsequent differences.	Yao et al in a meta-analysis noted that skin incision for the mini subvastus approach was significantly shorter than the conventional group.	Yao et al found a longer duration of surgery in mini subvastus approach compared with the conventional medial parapetallar.
Bonutti et al reported no difference between midvastus and subvastus approaches	Peng et al found improvements in ROM at 1 wk and 12 mo in the mini subvastus group. However, there were no differences thereafter.	Bourke et al found no differences with respect to long-term clinical benefits between medial parapatellar arthrotomy or the subvastus approach.	Kye-Youl Cho et al meta-analysis reported the length of the skin incision was significantly shorter in the MIS group compared with the limited medial parapatellar group.	Xu et al reported that MIS surgical techniques take longer then a conventional medial parapatellar arthrotomy
Kye-Youl Cho et al found that quadriceps force was stronger in the mini midvastus group when compared with the limited medial	Kye-Youl Cho et al found no difference comparing ROM between MIS and the limited medial parapatellar	Kye-Youl Cho et al found no statistical difference between the MIS or the limited medial parapatellar.	—	Li et al found also found longer surgical times in MIS.

(continued on next page)

Early vs Late Recovery	ROM	KS Scores	Length of Incision and Cosmesis	Duration of Surgery
parapatellar group at 6 wk				
Heekin and Fokin showed no clinical differences between the mini midvastus group and the limited medial parapatellar group	Xu et al who found increased ROM with mini midvastus approach in the first 2 wk only.	Nestor et al only found better quadriceps strength at 3 wk postoperatively between medial parapatellar arthrotomy and mini midvastus approaches.	—	—
Khakha et al reviewed MIS computer assisted TKA with conventional computer assisted TKA, and found early improvement in quadriceps strength and functional scores at 2 y with MIS but at 5 y there was no difference	—	Unwin et al found no difference in pain control or functional scores between MIS techniques and conventional approach.	—	
—	—	Kazarian et al only showed improved KSS from 1 to 3 mo postoperatively in the quadriceps-sparing group compared with the conventional approach.	—	—

Length of Hospital Stay	Radiographic Outcomes	Blood Loss	Pain Control	Wound Complications	Deep Vein Thrombosis
Obaid-ur-Rahman and Amin showed that length of say in the hospital was statistically shorter in the MIS group when compared with the traditional medial parapatellar (3.2–5.8 d)	Gandhi et al reported no difference in component or limb alignment when comparing MIS TKA with standard medial parapatellar approaches.	Peng et al showed no statistical differences between the quadriceps-sparing and standard groups with respect to blood loss.	Peng et al found a difference at 1 wk in VAS (−0.69) when comparing quadriceps-sparing patients with conventional approaches	Peng et al found no differences in wound complications between the quadriceps-sparing and conventional medial parapatellar approaches.	Peng et al in their meta-analysis found no differences in the incidence of DVT in the quadriceps-sparing group compared with the medial parapatellar group.
Peng et al showed no correlation between MIS quadriceps-sparing technique or conventional with respect to hospital length of stay.	Yuan et al revealed that the quadriceps-sparing approach has a risk of radiographic outliers. However, no definitive differences were found.	Yao et al reported no differences in blood loss comparing MIS with conventional.	Yao et al only found improvements at 1 and 3 d in the mini subvastus group compared with the conventional group	Li et al in a meta-analysis found an overall increase in wound healing complications in the MIS groups compared with the conventional medial parapatellar groups.	—
Yao et al found no difference in hospital stay when comparing the mini subvastus group with the conventional approach.	Yao et al in a radiographic analysis found no differences in hip–knee angle, femoral angle, tibial angle, femoral prosthesis flexion angle, and posterior slope angle of the tibial plateau in a comparison of the mini subvastus approach and medial parapatellar.	Kye-Youl Cho et al also found no difference in blood loss when comparing the mini midvastus with the limited medial parapatellar arthrotomy.	Xu et al meta-analysis found that pain control was improved in the early postoperative period (1–2 wk only) in the mini midvastus patients.	—	

(continued on next page)

Length of Hospital Stay	Radiographic Outcomes	Blood Loss	Pain Control	Wound Complications	Deep Vein Thrombosis
—	Kye-Youl Cho et al found no differences in radiographic outcomes when comparing mini midvastus group and the shortened medial parapatellar group	Li et al in a meta-analysis found a decrease in total blood loss in the MIS group when compared with medial parapatellar	—	—	—
—	Unwin et al found no radiographic differences at 6 y postoperatively between MIS approach and conventional approach.	—	—	—	—

Heekin and Fokin[16] further analyzed the comparison between the mini midvastus group and the limited medial parapatellar arthrotomy. They reported on 40 patients who underwent bilateral TKA with a limited medial parapatellar on one side and mini midvastus on the other side. Their findings showed no clinical differences between the approaches. They further went on to comment that the decision for choosing an approach should be based on the surgeon's comfort level.[16]

The possible advantages for MIS techniques in computer-assisted navigated cases have also been evaluated. Khakha and colleagues[17] reviewed the outcome comparing MIS computer assisted TKA with conventional computer assisted TKA, and they found an early improvement in quadriceps strength and functional scores at 2 years with the MIS approach, although at 5 years there was no difference.

Range of Motion

Several authors have attempted to identify potential benefits in postoperative ROM between the various MIS approaches. Obaid-ur-Rahman and Amin[18] found the ROM greater in patients who underwent a quadriceps-sparing approach. Yao and colleagues[14] also found early ROM improvements in their MIS group. At 1 and 3 days, patients in the mini subvastus group had improved ROM, but this normalized by 14 days postoperatively.

Peng and colleagues[19] were also able to display significant improvements in ROM at 1 week and 12 months in the mini subvastus group. However, all other follow-up visits before 1 year post operatively showed no difference as compared with the traditional approach. Cho and colleagues[15] found no difference when comparing ROM between the MIS approach and the limited medial parapatellar arthrotomy. These findings were also consistent with the results from the meta-analysis by Xu and colleagues,[20] who found significantly increased ROM with the mini midvastus approach in the first 2 weeks. However, after 2 weeks there was no difference in ROM. In summarizing all these reports, it seems that there may be an advantage to MIS approaches in the first few weeks after surgery, but by 3 months the ROM seems to be similar.

Knee Society Scores

Several studies have reviewed the functional outcomes between the traditional and MIS approaches. Obaid-ur-Rahman and Amin reported higher Knee Society (KS) scores in the quadriceps-sparing group when compared with the conventional approach at 1 and 3 months. Additionally, they found that patients who underwent a quadriceps-sparing approach were quicker to return to independent walking.[18] However, there were no differences in the functional KS scores after 3 months. A meta-analysis from Peng and colleagues[19] showed significant improvements in KS scores for the quadriceps-sparing group when compared with the conventional group at 3 months and 2 years. Yet, at 4 to 6 weeks there were no differences between the 2 groups. It is difficult to determine why there were increases in KS scores only at 3 months and then 2 years.

Conversely, Bourke and colleagues[21] compared outcomes on 90 patients undergoing bilateral TKA with either the standard medial parapatellar arthrotomy or the subvastus approach and found no differences with respect to long-term clinical benefits. They were only able to demonstrate better KS scores at 12 and 18 months. Similarly, when Cho and colleagues[15] reviewed KS functional scores, there was no statistical difference between the MIS or the limited medial parapatellar arthrotomy.

Nestor and colleagues[22] reviewed 27 patients undergoing bilateral TKA with the standard medial parapatellar arthrotomy or mini midvastus approach and found that the MIS approach had better quadriceps strength at 3 week postoperatively. No differences were found in any other outcome measures. Similarly, Unwin and colleagues[23] found that there was no difference in pain control or functional scores with their MIS techniques compared with the conventional approach. A meta-analysis from Kazarian and colleagues[24] showed improved KS scores at 1 to 3 months postoperatively in the quadriceps-sparing group compared with the conventional approach. After 3 months, no additional benefit was seen between the 2 groups. In reviewing these reported studies, we believe that the overall consensus shows no definitive improvement in KS scores when comparing MIS and conventional approaches.

Length of Incision and Cosmesis

There is an impression that a small skin incision with MIS TKA would be more appealing to patients. Although cosmesis is rather subjective, several authors have attempted to investigate the effect of the surgical approach on the skin incision. A meta-analysis by Smith and colleagues[25] demonstrated a significantly smaller length of the skin incision in the MIS groups. Lengths of incisions varied with each study ranging from 10 to 13 cm in the MIS groups and more than 13 cm in the conventional group. Additionally, they found greater ROM in the MIS; however, no other clinical or radiographic differences were seen. Yao and colleagues[14] noted that their skin incision for the mini subvastus approach showed to be significantly shorter than the conventional group. Cho and colleagues[15] reported the length of the skin incision was significantly shorter in the MIS group (9.6 cm) compared with the limited medial parapatellar group (11 cm). To our knowledge, no studies have evaluated the patients' perceptions of their surgical incisions.

Duration of Surgery

Many surgeons that have reservations toward MIS approaches have raised concerns about the potential for MIS to increase the operative time. Peng and colleagues[19] in a meta-analysis reported an increase in the duration of surgery. The mean difference in operative time between the MIS and standard approach was, on average, 18 minutes longer. Yao and colleagues[14] also compared the duration of surgery for the mini subvastus approach and the conventional medial parapatellar and they found the mini subvastus group had a significantly longer duration of surgery. Xu and colleagues[20] found an average increase of operative time of 11.64 minutes in the mini midvastus compared with medial parapatellar. The length of tourniquet time has also been seen in studies to be significantly longer in the mini midvastus group compared with the limited medial parapatellar group.[15] Other investigators have found that MIS techniques may take longer then a conventional medial parapatellar arthrotomy.[20,26]

Length of Hospital Stay

With the advent of rapid recovery programs and same-day TKA, there is a great deal of discussion of all aspects of patient care to improve unnecessary costs and added financial burden on the patient. Although many variables go into the length of stay, there have been some investigations into the surgical technique and surgical approach. Obaid-ur-Rahman and Amin[18] showed that length of say in the hospital was statistically shorter, 3.2 days in the MIS group when compared with 5.8 days in the traditional medial parapatellar group. Peng and colleagues,[19] conversely, showed no correlation between the MIS quadriceps-sparing technique or a conventional technique with respect to hospital length of stay. Likewise, Yao and colleagues[14] found no difference in hospital stay when comparing

the mini subvastus group with the conventional approach group. After reviewing the literature, surgical arthrotomy does not affect the length of stay after TKA.

Radiographic Outcomes

Accurate positioning of the components and limb alignment are paramount in TKA. The surgical approach should not jeopardize these parameters. A meta-analysis by Gandhi and colleagues[27] reported on complications between MIS TKA on standard medial parapatellar approaches and they found no difference in component or limb alignment. A meta-analysis by Yuan and colleagues[28] revealed that the quadriceps-sparing approach has a risk of radiographic outliers. compared with the conventional medial parapatellar approach, there were statistical differences in hip–knee angle, coronal tibial component angle, and femoral notch. No differences were seen with the coronal femoral angle. These radiographic outliers may certainly lead to component malalignment and malposition. Yao and colleagues[14] in a radiographic analysis found no differences in hip–knee angle, femoral angle, tibial angle, femoral prosthesis flexion angle, and posterior slope angle of the tibial plateau in a comparison of the mini subvastus approach and medial parapatellar arthrotomy. Comparably, other studies appreciated no differences in radiographic outcomes when comparing the mini midvastus group and the shortened medial parapatellar group.[15] Midterm data from Unwin and colleagues[23] echoed these findings at 6 years postoperatively with no differences in the radiographic alignment between their MIS approach and conventional approach. Overall, the literature shows no difference in radiographic outcomes between approaches.

COMPLICATIONS

Blood Loss

Reports have found consistent results with respect to blood loss when comparing MIS and standard approaches. Peng and colleagues[19] showed no statistical differences between the quadriceps-sparing and standard groups with respect to blood loss. This finding was also noted by Yao and colleagues.[14] Cho and colleagues[15] found no difference in blood loss when comparing the mini midvastus with the limited medial parapatellar arthrotomy. Conversely, Li and colleagues[26] in a meta-analysis found a decrease in total blood loss in the MIS group when compared with medial parapatellar. The majority of the literature shows no difference in blood loss when comparing MIS with conventional arthrotomies. Of note, in the meta-analyses, there was use of a tourniquet in the majority of studies. However, some never stated whether they used a tourniquet or not.

Pain Control

Peng and colleagues[19] found a difference at 1 week in visual analogue scale (VAS) scores when comparing quadriceps-sparing patients with conventional approaches. There was a decrease, on average, of 0.69 in VAS scores for the quadriceps-sparing group at the 1-week mark, but there were no differences at 4 to 6 weeks. Yao and colleagues[14] found that, at 1 and 3 days, patients in the mini subvastus group had improved VAS score when compared with the conventional group. However, this finding normalized in the subsequent days. Additionally, the mini subvastus cohort in the study by Peng and colleagues[19] displayed improved VAS scores for patients at the 1-year mark between compared with the conventional group.

Xu and colleagues[20] in a meta-analysis echoed theses findings and found that pain control was statistically improved (−0.20 VAS) in the early postoperative period (1–2 weeks) in the mini midvastus patients. However, no subsequent pain differences were seen on VAS scores after 2 weeks.

Wound Complications

With regard to incisional healing and infection rates, Peng and colleagues[19] found no differences in wound complications between the quadriceps-sparing and conventional medial parapatellar approaches. Similarly, no differences were demonstrated when comparing the mini subvastus group to the conventional group.[19] In contrast, Li and colleagues[26] in a meta-analysis found an overall increase in wound healing complications in the MIS groups compared with the conventional medial parapatellar groups. Although the literature shows no statistical difference, there may be a potential for wound healing complications.

Deep Vein Thrombosis

There are not many reports on the incidence of deep vein thrombosis with MIS approaches. However, Peng and colleagues[19] in a their meta-analysis found no differences in the incidence of deep vein thrombosis in the quadriceps-sparing group when compared with the medial parapatellar arthrotomy group.

SUMMARY

Throughout the history of TKA, we have continued to improve on the efficiency of the procedure. Even with the evolution of various MIS approaches, the traditional medial parapatellar approach remains a well-documented, successful surgical approach. No alternative approach to the knee has been able to successfully prove its superiority to the medial parapatellar. Nevertheless, many other TKA approaches have not been definitively found to be inferior to the conventional approach. This list includes the quadriceps-sparing, midvastus, subvastus, or limited medial parapatellar arthrotomies. All have been proven to be acceptable approaches when performing a TKA. The data available over the past 2 decades remain consistent regarding the comparison of MIS with conventional total knee approaches. There seems to be no definitive benefit to early postoperative function. Although some studies show a benefit in the first couple of weeks postoperatively, ultimately within the first few months the outcomes are comparable.[8,12,14–17]

When evaluating ROM, MIS techniques seem to have a potential advantage compared with the conventional approach. Some authors found a significant increase in ROM in the quadriceps-sparing and mini subvastus approaches. Still, this improvement seemed to only be present in the first few weeks after surgery.[15,18–20] Functional outcomes displayed a similar distribution of findings. Again, the MIS quadriceps-sparing technique has better improvement in KS scores in the immediate to early postoperative period; however, those results seemed to level out within the first 3 to 6 months postoperatively. Only 2 studies were able to show benefits in KSS scores beyond 1 year postoperatively.[15,18,19,21,22,24]

The length of the incision was very consistent across all studies. MIS techniques consistently proved to have smaller skin incisions compared with conventional groups. However, there seems to be no influence on surgical outcome. Additionally, to our knowledge there are no studies that examine patients' perception of their incisions while comparing approaches.[14,18]

Effects on the duration of surgery seem to be almost unanimous; most of the current literature available shows that the duration of surgery is prolonged with MIS techniques compared with traditional exposures. There are a few studies that contend these findings and report that there is no difference in surgical time. However, it should be noted that these reports were done in centers with a high volume by well-experienced surgeons.

Their findings, although valid, raise questions as to their reproducibility in lower volume institutions.[14,19,20,26]

Even with rapid recovery programs and same day TKA, there is no observed advantage to MIS approaches. Although some reports have shown a decreased length of stay with MIS approaches, others have reported no difference. Additionally, there seem to be many factors that influence a patient's length of stay and it is difficult to come to a consensus with many confounding variables at different institutions.[14,18,19]

With the introduction of MIS techniques, a valid concern was raised about the potential increase in radiographic outliers with the potential for early failure. With experience and meticulous technique, there is no difference in the incidence of radiographic outliers. However, Yuan and colleagues[28] cautioned surgeons on the potential risk for more outliers in the quadriceps-sparing approach.[14,23,27]

Overall, the use of both MIS and standard approaches prove to be acceptable in TKA. Neither has proved to be superior or inferior to the other. The decision to perform an MIS or standard approach remains with a surgeon's preference. With experience all techniques have been successful. Our recommendation is that surgeons choose a surgical approach that is most appropriate for the patient. Factors such as pathologic deformity, preoperative ROM, prior surgery and incisions, along with the diagnosis influence the chosen surgical approach. The outcome of TKA goes beyond the surgical approach.

DISCLOSURE

The authors have nothing to disclose.

REFERENCES

1. Long WJ, Hochfelder JP, Nett MP, et al. Insall & Scott Surgery of the Knee. 6th edition. 2019;149: 1652–64.e2.
2. von Langenbeck B. Zur resection des kniegelenke. Verh Dtsch En Geseuch F Chir 1879;7:23.
3. Insall J. A midline approach to the knee. J Bone Joint Surg Am 1971;53(8):1584–6.
4. Tria AJ, Scuderi GR. Minimally invasive knee arthroplasty: an overview. World J Orthop 2015; 6(10):804.
5. Tria AJ Jr, Coon TM. Minimal incision total knee arthroplasty: early experience. Clin Orthop Relat Res 2003;416:185–90.
6. Tria AJ Jr. Minimally invasive total knee arthroplasty: the importance of instrumentation. Orthop Clin North Am 2004;35(2):227–34.
7. Jackson G, Waldman BJ, Schaftel EA. Complications following quadriceps-sparing total knee arthroplasty. Orthopedics 2008;31(6):547.
8. Bonutti PM, Zywiel MG, Ulrich SD, et al. A comparison of subvastus and midvastus approaches in minimally invasive total knee arthroplasty. J Bone Joint Surg Am 2010;92(3):575–82.
9. Pagnano MW, Meneghini RM, Trousdale RT. Anatomy of the extensor mechanism in reference to quadriceps-sparing TKA. Clin Orthop Relat Res 2006;452(452):102–5.
10. Laskin RS, Beksac B, Phongjunakorn A, et al. Minimally invasive total knee replacement through a mini-midvastus incision: an outcome study. Clin Orthop Relat Res 2004;428:74–81.
11. Engh GA, Holt BT, Parks NL. A midvasus muscle-splitting approach for total knee arthroplasty. J Arthroplasty 1997;12(3):322–31.
12. Bourke MG, Buttrum PJ, Fitzpatrick PL, et al. Systematic review of medial parapatellar and subvastus approaches in total knee arthroplasty. J Arthroplasty 2010;25(5):728–34.
13. Aglietti P1, Baldini A, Sensi L. Quadriceps-sparing versus mini-subvastus approach in total knee arthroplasty. Clin Orthop Relat Res 2006;452: 106–11.
14. Yao Y, Kang P, Xue C, et al. A prospective randomized controlled study of total knee arthroplasty via mini-subvastus and conventional approach. Zhongguo Xiu Fu Chong Jian Wai Ke Za Zhi 2018;32(2): 162–8.
15. Cho K-Y, Kim K-I, Umrani S, et al. Better quadriceps recovery after minimally invasive total knee arthroplasty. Knee Surg Sports Traumatol Arthrosc 2014; 22(8):1759–64.
16. Heekin RD, Fokin AA. Mini-midvastus versus mini-medial parapatellar approach for minimally invasive total knee arthroplasty: outcomes pendulum is at equilibrium. J Arthroplasty 2014;29(2):339–42.
17. Khakha RS, Chowdhry M, Norris M, et al. Five-year follow-up of minimally invasive computer assisted total knee arthroplasty (MICATKA) versus conventional computer assisted total knee arthroplasty (CATKA)—a population matched study. Knee 2014;21(5):944–8.
18. Obaid-ur-Rahman, Amin. Less invasive versus standard total knee replacement: comparison of early outcome. J Pak Med Assoc 2015 Nov;65(11 Suppl 3):S82–6.
19. Peng X, Zhang X, Cheng T, et al. Comparison of the quadriceps-sparing and subvastus approaches versus the standard parapatellar approach in total knee arthroplasty: a meta-analysis of randomized controlled trials. BMC Musculoskelet Disord 2015; 16:327.
20. Xu SZ, Lin XJ, Tong X, et al. Minimally invasive midvastus versus standard parapatellar approach in

total knee arthroplasty: a meta-analysis of randomized controlled trials. PLoS One 2014;9(5):e95311.

21. Bourke MG, Jull GA, Buttrum PJ, et al. Comparing outcomes of medial parapatellar and subvastus approaches in total knee arthroplasty: a randomized controlled trial. J Arthroplasty 2012;27(3):347–53.

22. Nestor BJ, Toulson CE, Backus SI, et al. Mini-midvastus vs standard medial parapatellar approach: a prospective, randomized, double-blinded study in patients undergoing bilateral total knee arthroplasty. J Arthroplasty 2010;25(6 suppl):5–11.

23. Unwin O, Hassaballa M, Murray J, et al. Minimally invasive surgery (MIS) for total knee replacement; medium term results with minimum five year follow-up. Knee 2017;24(2):454–9.

24. Kazarian GS, Siow MY, Chen AF, et al. Comparison of quadriceps-sparing and medial parapatellar approaches in total knee arthroplasty: a meta-analysis of randomized controlled trials. J Arthroplasty 2018;33(1):277–83.

25. Smith TO, King JJ, Hing CB. A meta-analysis of randomised controlled trials comparing the clinical and radiological outcomes following minimally invasive to conventional exposure for total knee arthroplasty. Knee 2012;19(1):1–7.

26. Li C, Zeng Y, Shen B, et al. A meta-analysis of minimally invasive and conventional medial parapatellar approaches for primary total knee arthroplasty. Knee Surg Sports Traumatol Arthrosc 2015;23(7): 1971–85.

27. Gandhi R, Smith H, Lefaivre KA, et al. Complications after minimally invasive total knee arthroplasty as compared with traditional incision techniques: a meta-analysis. J Arthroplasty 2011; 26(1):29–35.

28. Yuan FZ, Wang SJ, Zhou ZX, et al. Malalignment and malposition of quadriceps-sparing approach in primary total knee arthroplasty: a systematic review and meta-analysis. J Orthop Surg Res 2017; 12(1):129.

Trauma

What's New in Percutaneous Pelvis Fracture Surgery?

Ishvinder S. Grewal, FRCS*,[1], Adam J. Starr, MD[1,2]

KEYWORDS

• Pelvis • Fracture • Percutaneous • Symphysis • Reduction • Fixation

KEY POINTS

- The percutaneous reduction and fixation of pelvic ring injuries is not a novel; posterior ring, anterior and posterior column fixation percutaneously is well-described and adopted as a safe technique.
- Pubic symphyseal disruptions are almost all exclusively treated with open reduction and internal fixation.
- There exists a growing body of evidence describing the percutaneous reduction and fixation of pubic symphysis injuries.
- Biomechanical comparisons between plate and screw fixations show little difference.
- Early clinical results of percutaneous symphysis fixation are promising.

INTRODUCTION

The treatment of pelvic and acetabular fractures with minimally invasive reduction techniques and percutaneous fixation is now a widely accepted method. Fixation of posterior ring injuries with iliosacral and trans-sacral screws is widely described, as is the use of anterior and posterior column screws and InFix anterior fixation. Various other screw corridors have been described and are accepted by certain centers as, at the very least, an adjunct to traditional open fracture management.

Posterior Ring

Percutaneous fixation of the posterior ring was first described in 1991 in small animals using a single trans-sacral screw.[1] The first published use of this technique in humans was the same year and used computed tomography-guided planning and intraoperative computed tomography-guided post wire insertion before drilling and screw insertion.[2] The first series in humans was published in 1995, recording the early outcomes and complications in 68 patients.[3] At the time, this was regarded almost as heresy; previously, these fractures had all been treated with large posterior approaches and open reduction and internal fixation having been described in 1976 by Letournel.[4] Although he himself states this was described twice prior, initially as early as 1913 by Lambotte.[5] Almost 25 years since Routt and Mayo published their early series, percutaneous fixation of the posterior ring is widely accepted as the standard of care in many institutions treating pelvic fracture and is described in the AO manual.[6]

Anterior Ring

Anterior column and ramus fractures are currently treated in a variety of ways. Either via open reduction and fixation via various anterior approaches, or percutaneous fixation with anterior column screws or the InFix method.

Retrograde superior ramus screws for the treatment of anterior pelvic ring disruptions were initially described by Lambotte and Tile[7]

Parkland Memorial Hospital, University of Texas Southwestern, 5201 Harry Hines Boulevard, Dallas, TX 75235, USA
[1]Present address: Parkland Health & Hospital System, 5200 Harry Hines Blvd, Dallas, TX 75235
[2]Present address: UT Southwestern Medical Center, 5323 Harry Hines Blvd, Dallas, TX 75390, USA
* Corresponding author. Parkland Health & Hospital System, 5200 Harry Hines Blvd, Dallas, TX 75235, USA
E-mail address: ISHI@DOCTORS.ORG.UK

Orthop Clin N Am 51 (2020) 317–324
https://doi.org/10.1016/j.ocl.2020.02.010
0030-5898/20/© 2020 Elsevier Inc. All rights reserved.

at the beginning of the 20th century,[8] but it was Routt and colleagues[9] in 1995 who advanced the technique into the mainstream. Percutaneous fixation of the columns was described by Starr and colleagues[10] in 1998. The first surgery performed in a 24-patient series, reported in 2002, occurred in 1991; this patient had undergone closed reduction and percutaneous fixation of an anterior column acetabular fracture.[11]

External fixation has long been a used as both temporary and definitive fixation of the anterior ring. As with any external fixation technique, the benefits include minimal invasivity, preservation of biology, decreases in operating time and blood loss, and technical ease. Disadvantages are the mechanical disadvantage of distance of pins to bone, low patient satisfaction in living with a pelvic external fixator, and risk of pin site infections and pin loosening, as well as a second surgery to remove the fixator.

Another described percutaneous method of fixation of the anterior ring is the InFix. The original description of the fixator was by Kuttner and colleagues,[12] who published an explanation of the surgical technique and midterm clinical results in the German literature in 2009. Vaidya and colleagues[13] described the modified method and introduced the nickname InFix in the English literature in 2012.

So one can see that percutaneous fixation of pelvic ring fractures is certainly not new, with these techniques all having been initially described more than 10 to 25 years ago. What has happened is that these techniques have now become accepted by the mainstream body of pelvic surgeons as acceptable and some would argue superior alternatives to open reduction and internal fixation.

WHAT'S NEW?

Following this is the question of what's new? What have we yet to achieve? We believe that currently the management of symphyseal injuries is still one that the overwhelming body of pelvic surgeons would still treat with open reduction and plating via a Pfannenstiel approach. This is because of the relative ease of accessibility to the anterior pelvic ring, good access to the surgical target, low incisional hernia rates,[14] and perceived low infection rates. This technique is not without its disadvantages though. The approach requires dissection through a complex anatomic region. Access for plate insertion often requires lateral incision extension, particularly in larger patients. This extension can increase the risk of damage to inguinal canal and its contents

and result in ongoing pain symptoms. The approach also sometimes requires the detachment of the distal insertion of the rectus abdomens muscles. The sequelae of this detachment were discussed by Pennal.[15] The vascular anatomy of the anterior pelvis is well-described and, although a surgeon familiar with this approach is aware of this anatomy, the risk of catastrophic hemorrhage by injury to the corona mortis should not be taken lightly. Finally, the risk of infection is certainly greater in obese[16,17] and diabetic patients.

Both anterior InFix and ex-fix can be used for the treatment of anterior pelvic ring injuries. Isolated symphyseal injuries though tend to be treated with open reduction and internal fixation. This is because an anatomic reduction and rigid fixation of the pubic symphysis is difficult to achieve through either InFix or ex-fix owing to the large distance from the fixation points to the symphysis. The benefit of anatomic reduction of the anterior ring is resultant improved alignment of posterior ring, allowing for easier posterior reduction and fixation.

PERCUTANEOUS SYMPHYSEAL FIXATION

This brings us to percutaneous fixation of the symphysis. In 2009, Mu and colleagues[18] described a series of patients with symphyseal injuries whom they treated with percutaneous screw inserted using navigation. They treated 8 patients over a 20-month period with a variety of ring injuries, including symphyseal injuries. Any patients in whom a closed or percutaneous reduction was not possible were excluded from the series and underwent standard open reduction and internal fixation. They reduced the symphysis with manual pressure on both iliums and then fine tuned the reduction with a percutaneously inserted clamp or towel-clip anteriorly.

They used navigation for screw insertion. The entry point of the screw was selected in the junctional zone between the pubic tubercle and superior ramus of pubis of either side. A 3.2 mm guidewire was inserted parallel to the superior border of the symphysis. Percutaneous drilling then occurred taking care to protect the spermatic cord in males.

Four OTA-AO B1 type fractures were treated with a single 7.3-mm cannulated screw. Two B2 and 2 C type fractures were treated with a second 7.3-mm screw from the base of the opposite pubic tubercle to the superior part of the contralateral pubic body. The reported mean blood loss was less than 10 mL and the mean surgical time was 57 minutes (range, 30–80 minutes).

They reported no complications and no losses of reduction.

Cano-Luis and colleagues[19] performed a biomechanical analysis of this new method of fixation, which they had been using in their institution for the treatment of Tile B1 and B3 fractures. They felt their intermediate clinical data were promising and therefore they performed a cadaveric biomechanical study. They used 2 × 6.5-mm crossed cannulated screws. They did not compare the strength of screw fixation with traditional fixation, but rather compared the displacement under load of 300N of an intact pelvis versus an injured pelvis that had undergone fixation. When they compared the symphysis of intact pelvises and injured pelvises that had been fixed, they found no difference in either the upper of lower symphysis under load.

Yao and colleagues[20] also carried out a biomechanical finite element study comparing 5 different methods of symphyseal fixation (Fig. 1). They did not place any posterior fixation in their models. Their results were certainly interesting. None of the 5 modes of fixation significantly restored overall construct stiffness. This finding perhaps confirms what is already practiced, in that we rarely fix the anterior ring without stabilizing the posterior ring also. Posterior fixation is also required in these injury patterns. What was interesting was that although single screw fixation lacked the stiffness of either single or dual plate fixation, dual screw fixation in either configuration was stiffer than both plating constructs.

Pelvic ring stability was assessed under 3 different loads and 3 displacement variables (Fig. 2). Under dual leg standing, parallel screw fixation showed the best fixation effect to horizontal displacement. In single-leg stance, the crossed screw model showed greater resistance to shear. Rotationally, the dual plate technique offered the greatest resistance to rotation. Obviously, this study is limited, but it shows that plate fixation is not necessarily superior to cannulated screw fixation in the symphysis.

Most recently, Yu and colleagues[21] published their retrospective case-control study comparing 24 Tile B1 patients treated with single percutaneous screw fixation with 27 who were treated with traditional open reduction and plating. They also performed biomechanical study with a 600N vertical central load. They found a lower maximal displacement with plating (0.408 mm), but displacement with a single screw was still only 0.643 mm. The previous studies have shown this can be improved upon greatly with the

addition of a second screw. Of greater importance, they showed a significant improvement in intraoperative blood loss, operative time, and length of scar in the percutaneous screw fixation group. There was no significant difference in preoperative or postoperative displacement, immediately postoperatively, at 3 months, or at final follow-up. There was no significant difference in implant failure, wound infection, or revision surgery.

Clearly, there is a justifiable fear of percutaneously instrumenting the structures at the front of the pelvis. However, a similar fear once existed around the posterior pelvic structures also. Pelvic surgery, whether open or percutaneous, is fraught with potential dangers, but these factors can be reduced with an understanding of the anatomy in the area. Ma and colleagues[22] performed a small cadaveric specimen study on 6 men and 2 women. They dissected out the spermatic cord, round ligament, and the corona mortis. They looked at the structures and their relationship to the bony structures. They found safe channels for both the insertion of parallel screws and crossed screws (Fig. 3).

The superior screw channel for the parallel technique has an entry point on the outer edge of the pubic tubercle and an exit point on the outer edge of the contralateral tubercle. They found a 4.5- or 6.5-mm screw was suitable for this channel. They also described safe channels for the second screw. For parallel fixation, the entry point was 20 mm lateral and 23 mm beneath the symphysis. The exit point was symmetric. This second channel was suitable for a 4.5-mm screw only.

For crossed screw fixation, they again started and exited 20 mm lateral to the symphysis, but exited 23 mm beneath the contralateral pubic symphysis. These screws were inserted at an angle of 25° to the horizontal and this channel allowed for only 4.5-mm diameter screws.

Having read this compelling literature, the senior author felt enough evidence existed to review the anatomy himself. As one can see from Figs. 4 and 5, there is a clear safe corridor avoiding key structures.

He then began using this technique. Thus far, the results have been promising enough that he has only performed 1 traditional open symphyseal fixation in the past 2 years. This patient was treated open because the senior surgeon was unable to successfully pass the guidewire across the correct channel despite several attempts. Ironically, this traditional fixation still failed! In the same time period he and his

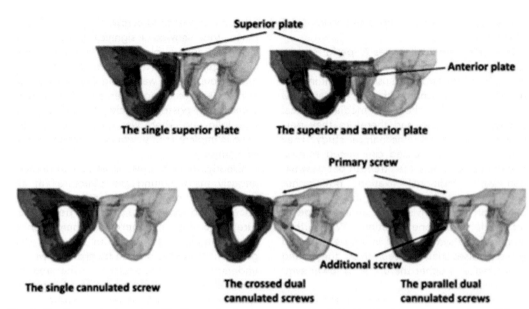

Fig. 1. Fixation methods analyzed by Yao and colleagues. (*From* Yao F, He Y, Qian H, et al. Comparison of Biomechanical Characteristics and Pelvic Ring Stability Using Different Fixation Methods to Treat Pubic Symphysis Diastasis: A Finite Element Study. Medicine (Baltimore) 2015;94(49):e2207; with permission.)

colleague have performed 30 procedures percutaneously.

We present one case that shows both the compelling indications and the reduction and fixation possible using these percutaneous techniques (**Fig. 6**). The patient is a 46-year-old unemployed active crack cocaine user who got into an altercation that led to him being run over twice. He sustained multiple injuries. Orthopedic injuries included a right bimalleolar ankle fracture, a left segmental femoral neck/shaft fracture, and a complex pelvic ring injury. He also had a bowel injury and a left common iliac artery injury with left lower limb ischemia. He

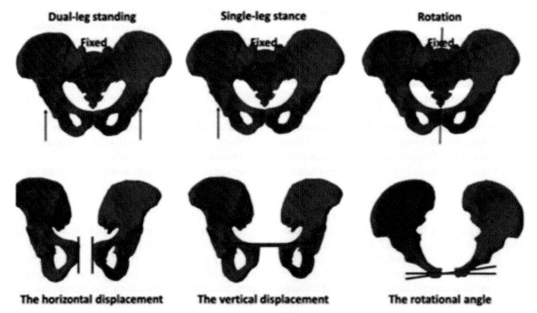

Fig. 2. Loading and displacement assessed by Yao and colleagues. (*From* Yao F, He Y, Qian H, et al. Comparison of Biomechanical Characteristics and Pelvic Ring Stability Using Different Fixation Methods to Treat Pubic Symphysis Diastasis: A Finite Element Study. Medicine (Baltimore) 2015;94(49):e2207; with permission.)

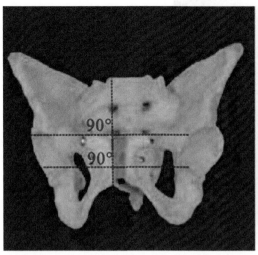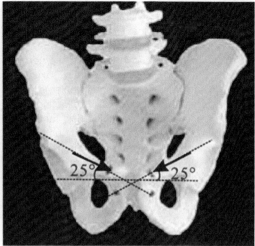

Fig. 3. Safe screw channel directions. (*From* Ma K, Zhu L, Fang Y. [A preliminary anatomical study on design of cannulated screw channels for fixation of symphysis pubis diastasis in small samples]. Zhongguo Xiu Fu Chong Jian Wai Ke Za Zhi 2014;28(1):43-6; with permission.)

underwent emergency stabilization of the pelvis via external fixator before having a diverting colostomy via laparotomy, iliac vessel stenting, and fasciotomies of left thigh and lower leg. He returned to the operating room the next day for left gluteal fasciotomies.

His pelvis ring injury included a right sacroiliac joint dislocation, left sacral fracture, and a diastased pubic symphysis. His fracture was vertically and rotationally unstable. He also had significant preexisting sacroiliac joint degenerative changes. He returned to the operating room 72 hours later for fixation of his femoral neck and shaft fracture and debridement of necrotic tissue from his abductors resulting from his vascular injury.

After an additional 72 hours he returned to the operating room for stabilization of his pelvic ring. This gentleman was very unwell medically, had open wounds on his buttock, thigh and leg, and a colostomy. Therefore, we believe, open surgery would have been risky.

As one can see from his intraoperative fluoroscopy images, his pubic symphysis was widely disrupted and unstable (Figs. 7 and 8). However, with knowledge of the local anatomy and use of a pelvic reduction frame, we performed a percutaneous reduction. Initially, we provisionally fixed the right sacroiliac joint and fixed the patient to the pelvic reduction frame. We then placed an external fixator pin into the symphysis and then used a motor to drive the pubis to a position of improved reduction (Figs. 9 and 10). We then applied a Weber clamp percutaneously across the disruption to further improve the reduction (Figs. 11 and 12). The key to safe application of the Weber percutaneously is an understanding of the local anatomy. As is shown in our diagrams, a safe zone exists between the spermatic cord and the neurovascular bundle. So long as the clamp is carefully introduced medial to the neurovascular bundle and lateral to the pubic tubercle the risk of injury to key structures is minimized. After this, we

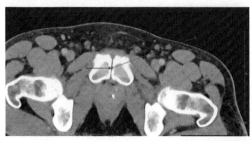

Fig. 4. Safe channel trajectory for screw insertion axial cross-section.

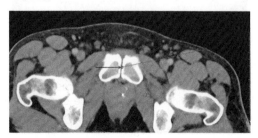

Fig. 5. Screw insertion: clamp placement safe zone.

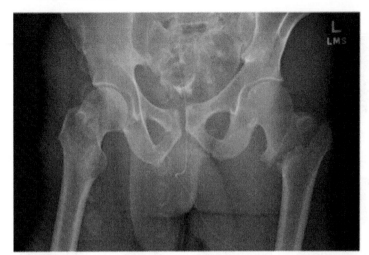

Fig. 6. Initial injury films in binder.

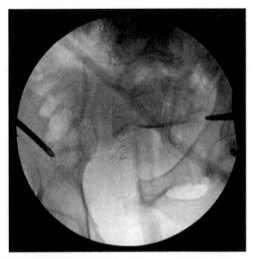

Fig. 7. Intraoperative fluoroscopy image showing widely disrupted symphysis.

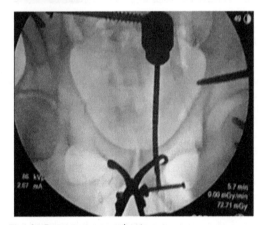

Fig. 9. Percutaneous reduction.

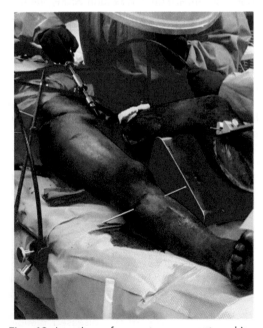

Fig. 8. Intraoperative inlet views.

Fig. 10. Insertion of percutaneous motor driven external fixator pin.

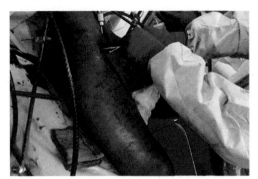

Fig. 11. Application of percutaneous Weber clamp.

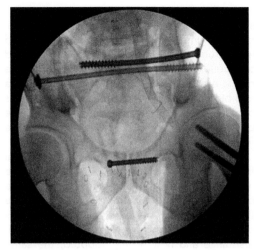

Fig. 14. Final anteroposterior fluoroscopy image.

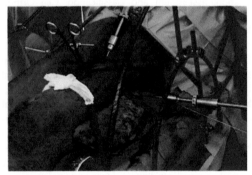

Fig. 12. Percutaneous reduction.

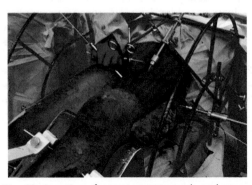

Fig. 13. Insertion of percutaneous symphyseal screw.

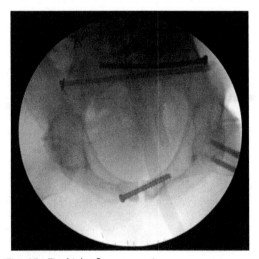

Fig. 15. Final inlet fluoroscopy image.

inserted a single 6.5-mm screw across the pubic symphysis (**Fig. 13**). We then fixed his bilateral posterior ring injuries, right sacroiliac joint, and left sacrum with iliosacral screws in the standard technique. A good reduction and fixation of the ring was achieved with minimal surgical trauma and blood loss (**Figs. 14** and **15**). We think this demonstrates both the ability to treat these percutaneously and also the patient subtype for whom it is almost certainly beneficial.

Percutaneous symphyseal fixation is the final frontier of percutaneous pelvic surgery. There remains a significant amount of work to be done to develop the instrumentation and hone the technique. We believe that just as previous percutaneous techniques were initially met with resistance and now widely adopted, the same will be true for this technique.

DISCLOSURE

The authors have nothing to disclose.

REFERENCES

1. Kaderly RE. Stabilization of bilateral sacroiliac fracture-luxations in small animals with a single transsacral screw. Vet Surg 1991;20(2):91–6.
2. Nelson DW, Duwelius PJ. CT-guided fixation of sacral fractures and sacroiliac joint disruptions. Radiology 1991;180(2):527–32.
3. Routt ML Jr, Kregor PJ, Simonian PT, et al. Early results of percutaneous iliosacral screws placed with the patient in the supine position. J Orthop Trauma 1995;9(3):207–14.
4. Letournel E. Pelvic fractures. Injury 1978;10(2):145–8.
5. Lambotte A. Chirurgie opératoire des fractures. Paris: Masson; 1913.
6. Website: AO Surgery Reference: iliosacral screw for SI joint. Available at: https://www2.aofoundation. org/wps/portal/surgerymobile?showPage=redfix& bone=Pelvis&segment=Ring&basicTechnique=Ili osacral%20screw%20for%20SI%20joint&backLink= both. Accessed January 8, 2020.
7. Tile M. Fracture of the pelvis and acetabulum. Baltimore (MD): Williams and Wilkins; 1984.
8. Cole PA, Dyskin EA, Gilbertson JA. Minimally-invasive fixation for anterior pelvic ring disruptions. Injury 2015;46(Suppl 3):S27–34.
9. Routt ML Jr, Simonian PT, Grujic L. The retrograde medullary superior pubic ramus screw for the treatment of anterior pelvic ring disruptions: a new technique. J Orthop Trauma 1995;9(1):35–44.
10. Starr AJ, Reinert CM, Jones AL. Percutaneous fixation of the columns of the acetabulum: a new technique. J Orthop Trauma 1998;12(1):51–8.
11. Crowl AC, Kahler DM. Closed reduction and percutaneous fixation of anterior column acetabular fractures. Comput Aided Surg 2002;7(3):169–78.
12. Kuttner M, Klaiber A, Lorenz T, et al. Neugebauer The pelvic subcutaneous cross-over internal fixator. Unfallchirurg 2009;112:661–9 [in German].
13. Vaidya R, Colen R, Vigdorchik J, et al. Treatment of unstable pelvic ring injuries with an internal anterior fixator and posterior fixation: initial clinical series. J Orthop Trauma 2012;26(1):1–8.
14. Cole JD, Bolhofner BR. Acetabular fracture fixation via a modified Stoppa limited intrapelvic approach. Description of operative technique and preliminary treatment results. Clin Orthop Relat Res 1994;(305):112–23.
15. Pennal GF, Tile M, Waddell JP, et al. Pelvic disruption: assessment and classification. Clin Orthop Relat Res 1980;(151):12–21.
16. Sems SA, Johnson M, Cole PA, et al, Minnesota Orthopaedic Trauma Group. Elevated body mass index increases early complications of surgical treatment of pelvic ring injuries. J Orthop Trauma 2010;24(5):309–14.
17. Purcell KF, Bergin PF, Spitler CA, et al. Management of pelvic and acetabular fractures in the obese patient. Orthop Clin North Am 2018;49(3):317–24.
18. Mu WD, Wang H, Zhou DS, et al. Computer navigated percutaneous screw fixation for traumatic pubic symphysis diastasis of unstable pelvic ring injuries. Chin Med J 2009;122:1699–703.
19. Cano-Luis P, Giráldez-Sanchez MA, Martínez-Reina J, et al. Biomechanical analysis of a new minimally invasive system for osteosynthesis of pubis symphysis disruption. Injury 2012;43(Suppl 2): S20–7.
20. Yao F, He Y, Qian H, et al. Comparison of biomechanical characteristics and pelvic ring stability using different fixation methods to treat pubic symphysis diastasis: a finite element study. Medicine (Baltimore) 2015;94(49):e2207.
21. Yu KH, Hong JJ, Guo XS, et al. Comparison of reconstruction plate screw fixation and percutaneous cannulated screw fixation in treatment of Tile B1 type pubic symphysis diastasis: a finite element analysis and 10-year clinical experience. J Orthop Surg Res 2015;10:151.
22. Ma K, Zhu L, Fang Y. A preliminary anatomical study on design of cannulated screw channels for fixation of symphysis pubis diastasis in small samples. Zhongguo Xiu Fu Chong Jian Wai Ke Za Zhi 2014;28(1):43–6 [in Chinese].

Minimally Invasive Treatment of Displaced Intra-Articular Calcaneal Fractures

Brandon G. Wilkinson, MD, John Lawrence Marsh, MD*

KEYWORDS

- Displaced intra-articular calcaneal fractures • Minimally invasive • Limited approach
- Percutaneous reduction

KEY POINTS

- Outcomes of minimally invasive surgical techniques are well documented and show good articular reductions and functional outcomes and have a very low incidence of wound complications and surgical site infections.
- Minimally invasive techniques can be applied broadly but have particular advantages in patients with higher than usual risk to soft tissues.
- Early timing for surgery plays a role in the effectiveness of minimally invasive surgery as mobile fracture fragments and ligamentotaxis are crucial to the success of indirect reduction and fixation.

INTRODUCTION: NATURE OF THE PROBLEM

There are very few fractures that have precipitated such debate about treatment as the displaced intra-articular calcaneus fracture (DIACF). DIACFs result from high-energy trauma, and surgical treatment requires understanding of the complex calcaneal anatomy and fracture characteristics, and high regard must be placed on associated soft tissue injury for optimal surgical outcomes. The best surgical treatment techniques have been the topic of debate for several decades and remain controversial. The goals of any operative reduction and fixation technique are the same: restoration of subtalar joint congruence, Bohler angle, calcaneal height, alignment, and width while minimizing the chances for soft tissue complications. The fundamental basis of different treatments hinge on how much weight to place on achieving the fracture reduction goals versus the goals of avoiding further soft tissue compromise and complications.

Extensile lateral approaches for open reduction and internal fixation have been used, as this approach allows the fracture to be directly reduced and the fracture fragments in the posterior facet to be visualized. However, extensile approaches are often complicated by high rates of wound breakdown and infection.[1–7] In efforts to avoid soft tissue complications and preserve blood supply, innovative less-invasive techniques have been developed targeting reducing and fixing the joint while minimizing further damage to the soft tissue envelope. In broad terms, these techniques include minimally invasive percutaneous stabilization with pins/screws, arthroscopic-assisted reduction and internal fixation, and limited incision sinus tarsi open reduction and internal fixation.

Department of Orthopedics and Rehabilitation, University of Iowa Hospitals and Clinics, University of Iowa, 200 Hawkins Drive, Iowa City, IA 52242, USA
* Corresponding author.
E-mail address: j-marsh@uiowa.edu

Orthop Clin N Am 51 (2020) 325–338
https://doi.org/10.1016/j.ocl.2020.02.007

INDICATIONS/CONTRAINDICATIONS

Indications for surgical treatment of calcaneal fractures depend on the fracture pattern, degree of displacement, characteristics of the patient, and the patient's preferences. Fracture patterns with large fragments and wide displacement are ideal for treatment. These are patterns in which there is substantial opportunity to improve the position and obtain solid fixation. Minimally displaced fractures have good outcomes without surgery and extensively comminuted fractures present challenges for any technique of surgical treatment.

Patient characteristics are always important, and elderly patients with decreased activity levels and patients who have diabetes or are smokers are not good candidates for surgery. Percutaneous approaches are safer than extensile open reduction and therefore can be chosen for a wider range of patient risk profiles. In addition to avoiding further soft tissue compromise, minimally invasive techniques may also be favored in the multiply comorbid or tenuous trauma patient, or in patients with diabetes, peripheral vascular disease, obesity, or smokers who are baseline susceptible to poor wound healing. It must be noted, however, that timing may play a role in the effectiveness of minimally invasive surgery, as mobile fracture fragments and ligamentotaxis are crucial to the success of indirect reduction and fixation.

Patient preferences should always be considered in the decision to operate. The evidence supports that the differences in outcomes between operative and nonoperative techniques are narrow enough that patients should be given a choice on whether to intervene. When this is done, some patients will choose nonoperative treatment.

MINIMALLY INVASIVE TECHNIQUES
Percutaneous Reduction and Screw Fixation (Authors' Preferred Method)
Some investigators advocate avoiding any incisions other than percutaneous puncture wounds to minimize soft tissue injury. The reduction is entirely judged using fluoroscopy. The reduction is performed using percutaneously inserted instruments to control, lever, and apply traction to displaced fragments all with the goal of correcting calcaneal varus, calcaneal pitch, lateral displacement, and elevation of the depressed posterior facet. Fixation is performed using a wide variety of devices including Kirschner wires (K-wires), Steinmann pins, external fixator, and cannulated and noncannulated screws. The

evidence shows that reasonable reductions can be obtained and maintained using these techniques. For instance, Stulik and colleagues[8] showed excellent reduction (less than 2 mm articular displacement), low wound complications, and good functional outcomes using closed reduction and K-wire fixation and with a mean follow-up of 43.4 months. A comparative study (by the senior author (JLM) of this article) between the extensile lateral and minimally invasive percutaneous approach assessed 125 patients with intra-articular calcaneus fractures. There was no difference in the Bohler angle, loss of fracture reduction at fracture healing, need for late subtalar fusion, and implant removal. However, this study showed a consistent theme: there was a significant decrease in soft tissue complications in the group treated with minimally invasive percutaneous screw fixation.[9]

Arthroscopic Assisted Reduction and Internal Rotation
To directly visualize the intra-articular fracture lines, minimize soft tissue injury, and preserve blood supply, arthroscopic assisted reduction and internal fixation has been proposed by some investigators. Sivakumar and colleagues[10] showed that a combination of arthroscopic and percutaneous reduction techniques resulted in 87.5% of cases with less than 2 mm articular congruity postoperatively and favorable results compared with prior literature. Advocates for arthroscopic assistance find significant advantages of continuous monitoring of the subtalar joint, improvement of subtalar joint reduction, accessibility for joint debridement, removal of loose osteochondral fragments, and identifying screw penetration into the joint.[10–13] Caution must be used because the fluid necessary to maintain the ability to directly visualize the fracture may lead to increased soft tissue swelling from fluid extravasation. In addition, there is significant technical difficulty and potential for increased surgical time and added costs that should not be overlooked.

Limited Open Sinus Tarsi Approach
Limited open sinus tarsi approach has been proposed to limit soft tissue dissection while still allowing fracture reduction/plate stabilization. This technique requires a small 2-cm to 4-cm sinus tarsi incision to directly visualize the posterior facet and anterior lateral fragments to assist optimal fracture reduction. With this technique, a specially contoured plate is often inserted through the incision to obtain fixation.

Kikuchi and colleagues[14] showed that the Bohler angle was successfully restored and calcaneal width was narrowed with low soft tissue complication rates. Nosewicz and colleagues[15] showed good joint reduction and no loss of reduction at final follow-up on computed tomography scans by use of a mini open sinus tarsi approach. In a randomized controlled trial, Xia and colleagues[16] compared the extended lateral approach with limited sinus tarsi and percutaneous plate fixation. Their results showed decreased surgical times and fewer wound complications in the sinus tarsi approach. Most importantly, functional scores and radiographic parameters were equivalent at final follow-up. These findings have been corroborated by many other studies in the literature.[17–19]

SURGICAL TECHNIQUE/PROCEDURE
Authors' Preferred Surgical Technique
Minimally invasive percutaneous reduction and screw fixation.

Preoperative Planning
Thorough planning with assessment of fracture characteristics with appropriate imaging are crucial to intervene successfully. Adequate imaging of the calcaneus including lateral, Broden, and hindfoot view are imperative for understanding of the fracture characteristics and displacement. These images will be used fluoroscopically during the procedure so understanding them ahead is critical. Contralateral calcaneus films will be of help during intraoperative determination of restoration of calcaneal pitch, Bohler angle, and confirm surgical restoration of calcaneal height and alignment to the contralateral side. Advanced imaging with computed tomography scans in semi-coronal and axial planes increases the ability to understand the fracture fragments. Some surgeons also use 3-dimensional images.

Expedited operative intervention is necessary with preference within 7 to 10 days to ensure fragment mobility, as closed manipulation of fracture fragments through the percutaneous approach becomes increasingly difficult with longer delays. Indirect fracture reduction after 2 weeks is difficult through the authors' preferred technique. Given minimal soft tissue insult with this technique, swelling and ecchymosis should not disqualify a patient from early intervention with this technique.

Patient Positioning/Approach/Procedure
There are 4 essential steps to the percutaneous approach, including the following:

- Correct patient positioning and fluoroscopy
- Percutaneous fracture reduction
- Percutaneous noncannulated screw fixation
- Postoperative care

Step 1: Correct Patient Positioning on Fluoroscopy
Patient positioning and ensuring the ability to obtain clear fluoroscopic views are imperative to this approach:

- The patient is placed in the lateral decubitus position on a radiolucent operative table with a long foot overhang (Maquet or 4085 bed) accommodating for large C-arm access. The well-leg is positioned down and anterior, with the operative extremity posterior and elevated on a ramp of firm blankets or Bone Foam ensuring a perfect lateral position of the operative foot and ankle. The operative extremity is subsequently prepped with ChloraPrep scrub, and draped with a down drape, impervious "sticky U" drape, and 2 large U extremity drapes. The operating surgeon is positioned posterior to the patient enabling optimal position for fracture reduction and screw placement (**Fig. 1**).
- Three basic fluoroscopic views are required to do this procedure. Fluoroscopic views should be confirmed before prepping and draping of the

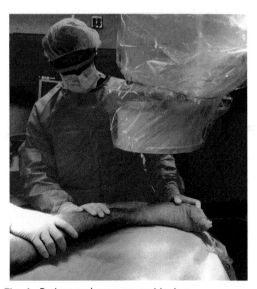

Fig. 1. Patient and surgeon positioning.

patient. Positioning the fluoroscopy unit angling in approximately 45° from the anterior and caudal aspect of the patient affords easy access to the lateral, lateral oblique (Broden) view, with fluoroscopy in the vertical position (Figs. 2 and 3).

- Visualization of the subtalar joint is best obtained by the lateral oblique view (see Fig. 3) with the C-arm rolled back approximately 30° with slight cant toward the foot of the bed. Posterior facet and subtalar joint visualization can further be fine-tuned by differing amounts of rotation and canting. With the fluoroscopy unit angled 45° to the foot of the bed, easy access to the hindfoot view (Harris view) (Fig. 4) is obtained by rolling the fluoroscopy unit back and beneath the corner of the table to the horizontal position with the surgeon holding the foot in dorsiflexion. These simple movements of the C-arm allow excellent views of the calcaneus and subtalar joint without need for manipulation of the foot or leg, which can potentially compromise provisional reduction and fixation throughout the procedure.

Step 2: Percutaneous Fracture Reduction
Percutaneous techniques for both joint depression and tongue-type calcaneal fractures are discussed separately, as they are different entities and require different reduction techniques.

Tongue-type fractures

- Two large (4-mm) threaded Steinmann pins are used for reduction of the posterior tuberosity fragment. The Steinmann pins are placed parallel from posterior into the facet fragment taking care to avoid the Achilles insertion and angled anteriorly in line with the fragment deformity (Fig. 5A). They should be advanced inferior to and to the level of the distal portion of the displaced facet on the tongue fragment. When seen on the Harris view, the Steinmann pins will be aligned parallel and in the central body of the calcaneus spaced by approximately 2 to 3 cm (Fig. 5B and C).

- Using the inserted Steinmann pins, the posterior fragment is reduced with downward pressure, valgus, and apposition of the fragment firmly against the articular surface of the talus (Fig. 6). A hemostat is often used under the anterior portion of the fragment, lifting it, to facilitate this reduction. Through this maneuver, the posterior facet is reduced, which also reduces the small tuberosity fragment, eliminating the need for manipulation of this fragment separately. The medial wall should be reduced. When the facet fragment is a tongue-type, the tuberosity fragment is small. Provisional fixation is with long K-wires inserted into the anterior calcaneus under fluoroscopic control. Occasionally, the Steinmann pins are inserted into the talus when there is inadequate anterior calcaneal bone to hold the tuberosity reduction. This happens in the setting of exceptionally large tongue-type fractures. The Steinmann pins can be left in place for several weeks for fractures with significant displacement. Screw fixation is described later in this article.

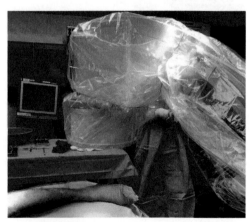

Fig. 2. Lateral view.

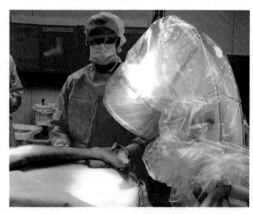

Fig. 3. Lateral oblique (Broden) view.

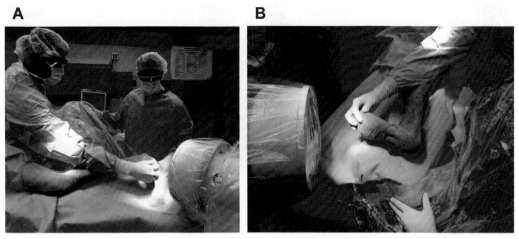

Fig. 4. (A) Fluoroscopy in the horizontal position to obtain the hindfoot (Harris) view. (B) Hindfoot view. Surgeon aids in view by dorsiflexing the patient's ankle.

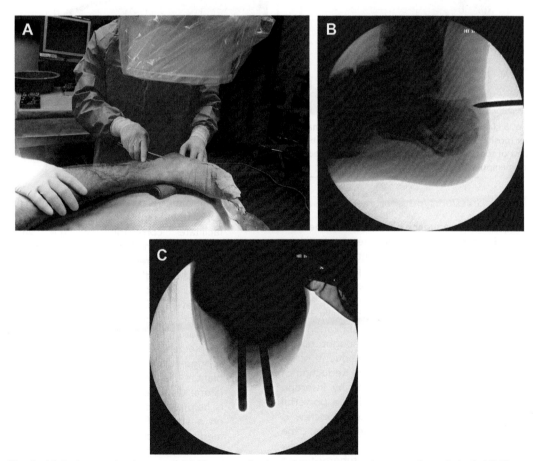

Fig. 5. (A) Steinman pin placement. (B) Fluoroscopic view of Steinman pin placement (lateral view). (C) Fluoroscopic view of Steinman pin placement (hindfoot view).

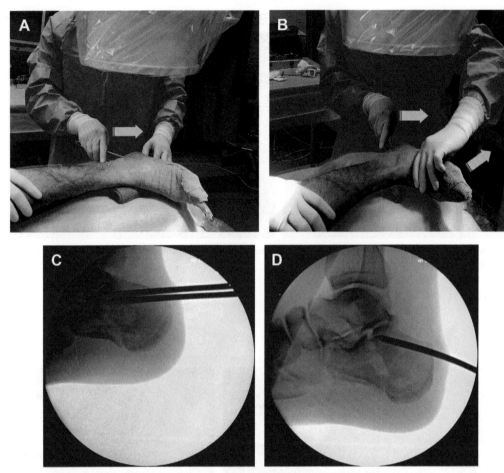

Fig. 6. (*A*) Tongue-type tuberosity reduction maneuver (position 1). (*B*) Tongue-type tuberosity reduction maneuver (position 2). (*C*) Fluoroscopic view of tongue-type tuberosity reduction maneuver (position 1). (*D*) Fluoroscopic view of tongue-type tuberosity reduction maneuver (position 2). *Yellow arrows* indicate direction of surgeon force for manipulation of fragments.

Joint depression type fractures

- Correct sequence of reduction maneuvers is necessary to obtain adequate articular reduction. It is important to note that you cannot reduce the posterior facet without first reducing the tuberosity as the first step in the procedure, as the displaced tuberosity is physically in the way. In addition, provisional fixation with K-wires should be well thought out in efforts to not block subsequent screw paths for definitive fixation. Reduction of the tuberosity is facilitated by insertion of a large corkscrew used as a powerful tool for manipulation. The corkscrew is placed lateral to medial in the tuberosity. Insertion of the corkscrew should be posterior in the tuberosity and centered in the anterior and posterior dimension. It is helpful to angle the corkscrew slightly superior to help facilitate correction of the varus deformity of the hindfoot (Fig. 7A–D).

- With a corkscrew properly inserted, and using the hindfoot view, manipulate the tuberosity out to length, correct varus and lateral displacement by posterior directed force, valgus and medial pressure (Fig. 7E). This maneuver can be supplemented by placing a laparotomy sponge at the base of the corkscrew and plantar flexing the ankle. To reduce lateral displacement of the tuberosity, it is helpful to place the medial malleolus on a stack of firm towels to allow for medial directed pressure on the tuberosity fragment with the corkscrew. Tilting the corkscrew into valgus will correct the varus deformity, as judged

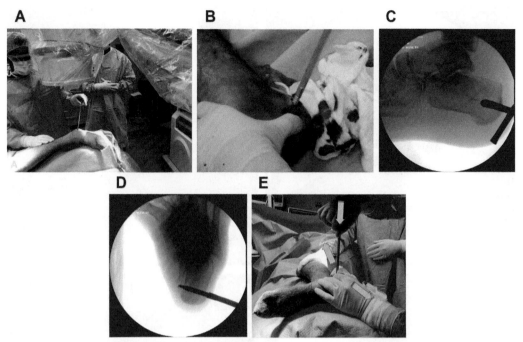

Fig. 7. (A) Corkscrew insertion. (B) Corkscrew insertion illustrating slight superior angulation on insertion. (C) Fluoroscopic view of corkscrew insertion (lateral view). (D) Fluoroscopic view of corkscrew insertion (hindfoot view). (E) Arrows indicate reduction forces applied by the surgeon. The surgeon places a laparotomy sponge at the base of the corkscrew to assist in distraction. With a combination of distraction, medially directed force, and valgus, the surgeon corrects length, lateralization, and varus malalignment of the calcaneus.

by the tuberosity medial wall alignment on the Harris view (see Fig. 7C). Occasionally it is requisite to use a small Cobb elevator or a hemostat inserted from a small lateral incision and navigated through the fracture fragments to manipulate the medial sustentaculum and translate the tuberosity against the instrument (a shoehorn type of technique) if the preceding measures are inadequate.

- The reduced tuberosity fragment as confirmed by fluoroscopic views is subsequently provisionally fixed with multiple K-wires (minimum of 3) placed medially and inferior in the tuberosity and efforts to not block subsequent reduction of the facet fragments. K-wire placement and reduction is again confirmed on fluoroscopic views.

- With the posterior tuberosity reduced and provisionally fixed with K-wires, reduction of the articular facet fragment is done using the lateral and lateral oblique views as the working views. The facet fragment is then reduced with superior directed pressure with a

laterally inserted curved hemostat placed directly beneath the rotated facet fragments (Fig. 8). If facet fragment mobilization is difficult, this is likely due to an inadequately reduced tuberosity fragment and confirmation of tuberosity fragment reduction should be revisited. With fluoroscopic confirmation of facet fragment reduction, 0.45-mm K-wires are subsequently used for provisional fixation. These K-wires should be placed lateral to medial, beginning slightly posterior and inferior to the distal fibula with the goal of capturing the reduced facet fragment and fixing it to the intact medial sustentaculum (see Fig. 8D). Adequate pin placement and facet reduction maintenance is confirmed on the lateral and lateral oblique views of the subtalar joint.

Step 3: Percutaneous Noncannulated Screw Fixation

Percutaneous screw fixation is used for definitive fixation of the reduced facet and tuberosity fragments. Screw start points, as well as final screw placement, should be well visualized and

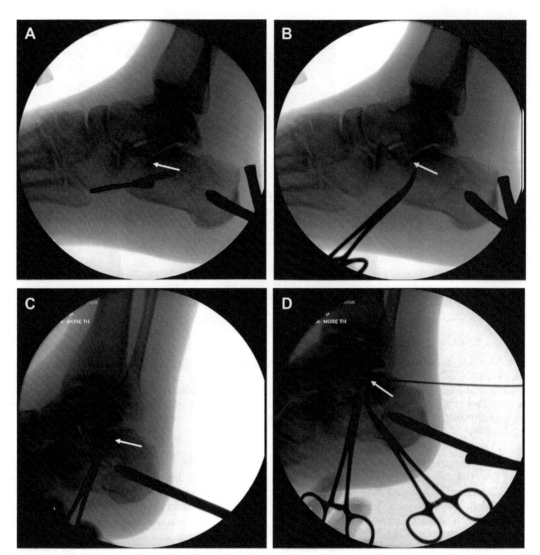

Fig. 8. (*A*) Curved hemostat is used to elevate the articular surface (*white arrow* illustrating unreduced position). (*B*) Yellow arrow illustrating the reduced position after hemostat manipulation. (*C*) Hemostat reduction of articular surface on lateral oblique view (*white arrow* illustrating facet in unreduced position). (*D*) Hemostat manipulation leads to reduced facet (*yellow arrow*) and provisional fixation with K-wire.

confirmed on all fluoroscopic views to ensure proper placement and avoidance of joint penetration. The authors prefer noncannulated screws, as the drill bit provides superior tactile feedback facilitating appropriate screw trajectory and then placement:

- The facet fragment is addressed first using 3.5-mm or 4.0-mm partially threaded noncannulated screws. As mentioned previously, the tactile feedback of the 2.5-mm drill is particularly helpful in identifying entrance into the sustentacular piece, as well as minimizing breach of the medial

wall and possible injury to the flexor hallucis longus tendon. Partially threaded screws with usual length of 35 to 45 mm are placed from lateral to medial capturing the facet fragment and compressing it to the sustentacular fragment (**Fig. 9**). The lateral view facilitates correct screw entry point, while the lateral oblique view allows accurate navigation of the screw into the sustentaculum. Screw length is best depicted with use of the hindfoot view.
- The tuberosity is then fixed with long fully threaded 3.5-mm screws (minimum of 2, maximum of 4 screws) (**Fig. 10**). It is

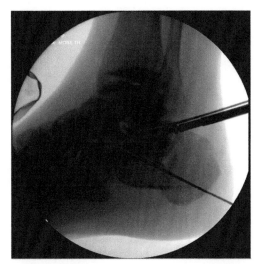

Fig. 9. Screw fixation of the facet fragment. Note the K-wire positioned to next fix the tuberosity fragment into the medial sustentaculum.

imperative that the screws fix the tuberosity fragment to both the medial sustentaculum as well as the anterior process of the calcaneus and, as such, multiple fluoroscopic views are necessary for correct screw placement. In general, 65-mm to 85mmm screw lengths are used and inserted using a power driver. The screws are inserted from posterior lateral in the tuberosity directed slightly superior and medial to engage the sustentaculum. In contrast to the facet fragment, the length of screws for the tuberosity fragment are best judged on the lateral view. Care should be taken to avoid medial sustentacular breech, as well as a prominent screw head on the tuberosity fragment to limit potential damage to the flexor hallucis longus tendon and dissatisfaction with prominent screw heads once swelling resolves.

- In tongue-type fractures, many similar screw paths are used. It is important the tongue fragment is well fixed. Anterior screws beneath the posterior facet into the sustentaculum secure the front of the tongue, and long screws from the back of the tongue fragment to the front of the calcaneus are needed. Screws also may be directed from the top of the tongue into the bottom of the calcaneus. In these cases, additional fixation can be achieved with inferiorly directed cancellous screws compressing the tongue fragment with the posterior tuberosity fragment.
- Diligent fluoroscopy using the lateral, oblique lateral, and hindfoot views should be used to confirm all screw positions and lengths, as well as maintenance of fracture reduction before leaving the operating room.

Step 4: Postoperative Care

- The operative extremity is placed in a short leg plaster splint with awareness of

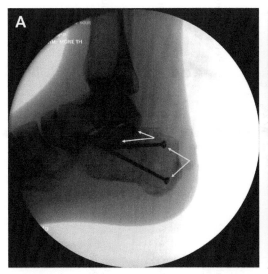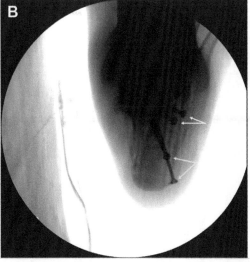

Fig. 10. Screw fixation of facet and tuberosity fragments on (*A*) lateral view and (*B*) hindfoot view. White and yellow arrows indicate facet screws and tuberosity screws respectively.

Table 1
Summary of results of limited minimally invasive approach techniques

Study, Year	Classification (Sanders)	Technique	Mean Age, y	% Female	Follow-up, mo	Outcomes
De Vroome & van der Linden,[20] 2014	Type II 28% Type III 56% Type IV 15%	Percutaneous	51	23	Not reported. Median follow-up 72 mo	AOFAS 69% good-excellent 31% fair-poor 100% tongue-type had good-excellent outcomes 2.4% infection rate
Tomersen et al,[21] 2011	Type II 26% Type III 39% Type IV 34%	Percutaneous	54	30	66	AOFAS 73% good-excellent 27% fair-poor
DeWall et al,[9] 2010	Type II 39% Type III 33% Type IV 6% Not specified 22%	Percutaneous	40	20	21.9	Average SF-36 score: 47.1 Foot Function index: 66.6 Deep infection 0% Superficial infection 6%
Walde et al,[22] 2008	Type II 16% Type III 57% Type IV 27%	Percutaneous	46	28	68	Zwipp score 61% good-excellent 39% fair-poor
Schepers et al,[23] 2007	Type II 38% Type III 28% Type IV 28%	Percutaneous	46	28	35	AOFAS 72% good-excellent 28% fair-poor
Stulik et al,[8] 2006	Type II 61% Type III 30% Type IV 9%	Percutaneous	44	15	43	Creighton-Nebraska Health Foundation Assessment score 72% good-excellent 28% fair to poor 1.7% deep infection rate

Study	Sanders Type	Procedure	No.		Follow-up	Outcomes
McGarvey et al,[24] 2006	Type II 33% Type III 27% Type IV 30%	Percutaneous + external fixation	42	23	25	AOFAS average score 66
Kikuchi et al,[14] 2013	Type II 36% Type III 32% Type IV 32%	Limited sinus tarsi	43	14	8	Restoration of Bohler angle and calcaneal width in all cases. 13.6% superficial infection.
Nosewicz et al,[15] 2012	Type II 9 Type III 13	Limited sinus tarsi + percutaneous screw fixation	45	14	32	No loss of reduction at final follow-up. AOFAS 86 Superficial wound infection 14%
Ebraheim et al,[25] 2000	Type II 67% Type III 23.6% Type IV 9.4%	Limited Sinus Tarsi + Percutaneous fixation	42	24	29	Mean AOFAS 77.6, Infection 8.5%
Xia et al,[16] 2014	Less invasive: Type II 66% Type III 42% Extensile lateral Type II 63% Type III 45%	Limited sinus tarsi vs extensile lateral	Less invasive: 38 Extensile Lateral: 37	Less invasive: 4 Extensile Lateral: 4	19	Decreased surgical time and wound complications in ST group. Maryland Foot Scores in ST group. No difference in radiographic parameters between groups.
Zhang et al,[17] 2014	Less invasive: Type II 46% Type III 33% Type IV 20% Extensile Lateral Type II 40% Type III 38% Type IV 22%	Limited sinus tarsi vs modified longitudinal approach	Less invasive: 40 Extensile Lateral: 41	Less invasive: 11 Extensile Lateral: 13	27	Decreased wound complications and operative time in less invasive group. Equivalent AOFAS scores.

(continued on next page)

Study, Year	Classification (Sanders)	Technique	Mean Age, y	% Female	Follow-up, mo	Outcomes
Kline et al,[18] 2013	Less invasive: Type II 61% Type III 39% Extensile Lateral Type II 53% Type III 47%	Less invasive vs extensile lateral	Less invasive: 46 Extensile lateral: 42	Less invasive: 21 Extensile lateral: 15	Less invasive: 28 Extensile lateral: 31	No difference in Foot Function index, VAS, or satisfaction rates. No difference in Bohler angle. Significant decrease in wound complications and secondary procedures in less-invasive group.
Weber et al,[19] 2008	Less invasive: Type II 83% Type III 17% Extensile lateral Type II 77% Type III 23%	Limited sinus tarsi vs extensile lateral	Less invasive: 43 Extensile: 40	Not reported	Less invasive: 31 Extensile: 19	Decreased surgical time in sinus tarsi group, equivalent functional outcomes. Increase ROH in sinus tarsi group.
Sivakumar et al,[10] 2014	Type II 56% Type III 22% Type IV 22%	ARIF	45	22	18	AOFAS 89% good-excellent. 11% fair-poor.
Woon et al,[11] 2011	Type II 100%	ARIF	43	22	24	Residual intra-articular incongruity less than 1 mm. Improvement in Medical Outcomes Study 36 SF, VAS, and AOFAS.
Gavlik et al,[12] 2002	Type II 100%	ARIF	40	15	14	No wound complications. AOFAS 93.7. No loss of reduction at final follow-up.

Abbreviations: AOFAS, The American Orthopedic Foot & Ankle Society; ARIF, Arthroscopic assisted Reduction and Internal Fixation; ROH, removal of hardware; SF-36, short form 36 question survey; VAS, visual analogue scale.

ankle alignment depending on the fracture type. To avoid undue stress on tongue-type injuries, the ankle is splinted and 20° of plantarflexion. Joint depression–type fractures are placed with the ankle in neutral alignment.

- Postoperative radiographs are performed to better visualize the final product. Computed tomography scans can additionally be used to further evaluate articular reduction and screw placement.
- The patient will return for a 2-week postoperative visit for a wound check and suture removal. Patients are then transitioned into a removable cast boot with physical therapy to begin active ankle and subtalar range-of-motion exercises. In cases of severely displaced fractures, the patient is transitioned into a short leg cast for 4 to 6 weeks. We recommend a total of 8 weeks of nonweightbearing for any operative calcaneus fracture.

OUTCOMES

Outcomes of treatment of DIACF with minimally invasive surgical techniques are well documented and a summary of results is listed in Table 1. The data show a very low incidence of wound complications, surgical site infections, and need for secondary procedures.[8,9,12,14–20,25] In addition, minimally invasive techniques have shown good results in restoration of the Bohler angle, articular congruity, and maintenance of reduction at final follow-up.[11,12,14,15,18] Perhaps most importantly, functional outcome scores are consistently good to excellent in patients treated with percutaneous or other minimally invasive techniques.[8–12,15–25]

SUMMARY

Minimally invasive surgical techniques are increasingly used for definitive treatment of displaced intra-articular calcaneal fractures. These approaches have been shown to minimize soft tissue injury, preserve blood supply, and decrease operative time. These methods can be applied to all calcaneal fractures and have particular advantages in patients with higher than usual risks to the soft tissues, such as smokers or patients with diabetes. Importantly, the literature suggests that results of limited soft tissue dissection approaches provide equivalent outcomes to those obtained with the extensile lateral approach, and an increasing number of surgeons are using these techniques for most or all DIACFs. The method of percutaneous reduction and screw fixation described in this article was developed by the senior author and has been his sole method of operative treatment of DIACF for more than 20 years. This technique requires relatively early surgery, which is crucial to successful percutaneous manipulation of fracture fragments. Debate remains about the optimal treatment of displaced intra-articular calcaneal fractures, but minimally invasive surgical techniques have been widely adopted by many surgeons. We predict that as imaging and other techniques continue to improve, more and more calcaneal fractures will be treated by these appealing safer techniques.

DISCLOSURE

B.G. Wilkinson: Nothing to Disclose. J.L. Marsh: Oxford Press, Biomet Trauma, Wright Medical – All Royalties.

REFERENCES

1. Abidi NA, Dhawan S, Gruen GS, et al. Wound-healing risk factors after open reduction and internal fixation of calcaneal fractures. Foot Ankle Int 1998;19:856–61.

2. Bibbo C, Ehrlich DA, Nguyen HM, et al. Low wound complication rates for the lateral extensile approach for calcaneal ORIF when the lateral calcaneal artery is patent. Foot Ankle Int 2014;35(7): 650–6.

3. Gardner MJ, Nork SE, Barei DP, et al. Secondary soft tissue compromise in tongue-type calcaneus fractures. J Orthop Trauma 2008;22(7):439–45.

4. Shuler FD, Conti SF, Gruen GS, et al. Wound-healing risk factors after open reduction and internal fixation of calcaneal fractures: does correction of Böhler's angle alter outcomes? Orthop Clin North Am 2001;32:187–92.

5. Buckley RE, Tough S. Displaced intra- articular calcaneal fractures. J Am Acad Orthop Surg 2004; 12(3):172–8.

6. Swanson SA, Clare MP, Sanders RW. Management of intra-articular fractures of the calcaneus. Foot Ankle Clin 2008;13(4):659–78.

7. Gougoulias N, Khanna A, McBride DJ, et al. Management of calcaneal fractures: systematic review of randomized trials. Br Med Bull 2009;92:153–67.

8. Stulik J, Stehlik J, Rysavy M, et al. Minimally invasive treatment of intra-articular fractures of the calcaneum. J Bone Joint Surg Br 2006;88:1634–41.

9. DeWall M, Henderson CE, McKinley TO, et al. Percutaneous reduction and fixation of displaced

intraarticular calcaneus fractures. J Orthop Trauma 2010;24(8):466–72.

10. Sivakumar BS, Wong P, Dick CG, et al. Arthroscopic reduction and percutaneous fixation of selected calcaneus fractures: surgical technique and early results. J Orthop Trauma 2014;28(10):569–76.

11. Woon CY, Chong KW, Yeo W, et al. Subtalar arthroscopy and fluoroscopy in percutaneous fixation of intra-articular calcaneal fractures: the best of both worlds. J Trauma 2011;71(4):917–25.

12. Gavlik JM, Rammelt S, Zwipp H. The use of subtalar arthroscopy in open reduction and internal fixation of intra-articular calcaneal fractures. Injury 2002; 33(1):63–71.

13. Beimers L, Frey C, van Dijk CN. Arthroscopy of the posterior subtalar joint. Foot Ankle Clin 2006;11: 369–90.

14. Kikuchi C, Charlton TP, Thordarson DB. Limited sinus tarsi approach for intraarticular calcaneus fractures. Foot Ankle Int 2013;34(12):1689–94.

15. Nosewicz T, Knupp M, Barg A, et al. Miniopen sinus tarsi approach with percutaneous screw fixation of displaced calcaneal fractures: a prospective computed tomography-based study. Foot Ankle Int 2012;33(11):925–33.

16. Xia S, Lu Y, Wang H, et al. Open reduction and internal fixation with conventional plate via L-shaped lateral approach versus internal fixation with percutaneous plate via a sinus tarsi approach for calcaneal fractures: a randomized controlled trial. Int J Surg 2014;12(5):475–80.

17. Zhang T, Su Y, Chen W, et al. Displaced intra-articular calcaneal fractures treated in a minimally invasive fashion: longitudinal approach versus sinus

tarsi approach. J Bone Joint Surg Am 2014;96(4): 302–9.

18. Kline AJ, Anderson RB, Davis WH, et al. Minimally invasive technique versus an extensile lateral approach for intra-articular calcaneal fractures. Foot Ankle Int 2013;34(6):773–8.

19. Weber M, Lehmann O, Sägesser D, et al. Limited open reduction and internal fixation of displaced intra-articular fractures of the calcaneum. J Bone Joint Surg Br 2008;90(12):1608–16.

20. De Vroome SW, van der Linden FM. Cohort study on the percutaneous treatment of displaced intra-articular fractures of the calcaneus. Foot Ankle Int 2014;35(2):156–61.

21. Tomersen T, Biert J, Frolke JP. Treatment of displaced intra-articular calcaneal fractures with closed reduction and percutaneous fixation. J Bone Joint Surg Am 2011;93:920–8.

22. Walde TA, Sauer B, Degreif J, et al. Closed reduction and percutaneous Kirschner wire fixation for the treatment of dislocated calcaneus frac- tures: surgical technique, complications, clinical and radiological results after 2-10 years. Arch Orthop Trauma Surg 2008;128:585–91.

23. Schepers T, Schipper IB, Vogels LM, et al. Percutaneous treatment of displaced intra-articular calcaneal fractures. J Orthop Sci 2007;12:22–7, 26.

24. McGarvey WC, Burris MW, Clanton TO, et al. Calcaneal fractures: indi-rect reduction and external fixation. Foot Ankle Int 2006;27:494–9.

25. Ebraheim NA, Elgafy H, Sabry FF, et al. Sinus tarsi approach with trans-articular fixation for displaced intra- articular fractures of the calcaneus. Foot Ankle Int 2000;21(2):105–13.

Pediatrics

Advances in Minimally Invasive Techniques in Pediatric Orthopedics
Percutaneous Spine Fracture Fixation

Ryan S. Bailey, MD, Aki Puryear, MD*

KEYWORDS

- Percutaneous pedicle screw • Pediatric • Spine • Fracture • Trauma • Fusionless instrumentation
- Internal brace

KEY POINTS

- There are situations when nonoperative treatment can be difficult or contraindicated secondary to other injuries, or patient factors.
- Temporary internal stabilization of pediatric spine fractures can provide good outcomes without traditional fusion techniques.
- Percutaneous pedicle screw instrumentation can be done safely with minimal soft tissue injury allowing for more physiologic healing than open procedures.

INTRODUCTION

Pediatric spine fractures are relatively rare and make up 2% to 5% of all spinal traumas.[1,2] Although these injuries are usually sustained via high-energy mechanisms and associated serious injury, nonoperative treatment is often the mainstay of treatment due to the significant healing and growth potential of the pediatric population.[3–5] There are several instances when nonoperative treatment is indicated, but cannot be used because of other injuries, such as chest and abdominal trauma, or patient factors, such as noncompliance or psychological disorders. When operative treatment is indicated secondary to the injury or when nonoperative treatment cannot be done because of other factors, traditional open instrumentation and fusion is less attractive due to risk of adjacent segment degeneration and the effects of spinal fusion on the growing spine. However, the growth and healing potential of the younger patents

allow less extensive treatment results similar results to adults.

Percutaneous pedicle screw instrumentation (PPSI) without fusion followed by subsequent removal of instrumentation is an option in the treatment of pediatric spinal fractures.[6] The technique allows earlier mobilization while acting as a mandatory internal brace, eliminating compliance, tolerance, and associated injury contraindications of bracing. PPSI has potential advantages over traditional open procedures, which include less blood loss and decreased postoperative pain.[7–12] Performing the procedure in a truly percutaneous manner, limiting exposing the periosteum and disrupting the facets, limits the risk of autofusion. Furthermore, instrumentation without fusion followed by later removal of instrumentation takes advantage of the high healing potential of the pediatric population and potentially preserves ultimate function and mobility of the spine not possible with fusion.

Department of Orthopaedic Surgery, Saint Louis University, 3635 Vista Avenue, 7th Floor-Desloge Tower, St Louis, MO 63110, USA
* Corresponding author.
E-mail address: aki.puryear@health.slu.edu

Percutaneous Pedicle Screw Instrumentation Technique

The surgical technique of PPSI uses the method of minimally invasive insertion of pedicle screws, rod fixation, and reduction of spinal injury. Specific factors such as fracture conditions, patient factors, and surgeon preference determine the exact steps, but generally follow the general pattern/approach described as follows.

Levels of stability are chosen for the appropriate stability of the fracture based on the number of levels, location, and fracture pattern. Most commonly, the chosen fixation includes 2 levels above and 2 levels below the injury.

The patient is positioned prone on a radiolucent operating table with the legs extended and the abdomen free of pressure. Fluoroscopy is used to identify the injured level(s), and the pedicle centers are located and marked both horizontally and vertically for all levels. Initial dissection is then carried out according to surgeon preference through either multiple small incisions or one longer midline incision (authors preference). Using a single midline incision, a superficial fascia exposure is performed for the insertion of percutaneous screws with minimal disruption of the soft tissue envelope.

Entry sites can be identified through O-arm or other imaging system assistance but are most commonly accomplished with the use of fluoroscopic guidance. Percutaneous screws are then placed by first cannulating the pedicles using Jamshidi needles. Using the anteroposterior (AP) fluoroscopic radiographs, the Jamshidi needle tip should be placed at the junction of the transverse process and the lateral facet joint. The needle is malleted into the bone approximately 2 cm without passing the medial wall of the pedicle on AP radiographic images. Positioning is then verified on lateral radiographic imaging and then advanced. Guidewires are then placed. The fascia is then incised, and the sites prepared using soft tissue sheaths that dilate the entry point while simultaneously protecting the muscle.

Screw lengths are measured, and the entry site prepared with an awl and a tap. Screws are then placed. The critical point of placement occurs when the screw head is buried on the superior facet, and all screw heights are verified at the same level of radiographic imaging. Once the position of all screws is confirmed, the rods are cut to an appropriate length and then placed subfacially into the screw heads. Appropriate reduction maneuvers, including ligamentotaxis and contouring, are used to aid in the reduction.

The most common maneuver is to compress the screw heads as an aid to reduction. Position, reduction, and placement of the rods are verified on fluoroscopic imaging.

Following final verification of the construct, the fascial, soft tissues, and skin are closed in a standard fashion. Depending on the injury and intraoperative findings, the surgeon may elect to close with or without placement of a drain. Postoperatively, an off-the-shelf soft brace is occasionally used for patient comfort. Mobilization is based on other injuries. If the spine is the only injury, a rapid mobilization protocol is used with patient up-to-chair on the first day, progression of walking and mobilization later in the day. Most patients meet discharge criteria by postoperative day 2 to 3. Patients are followed-up in 2 weeks for incision check. If a brace is used, it is recommended that the patient use it as needed for comfort. All implants are planned for removal between 6 and 12 months.

Outcomes

PPSI has been described extensively in the adult literature in recent years. Reports include its evolving use as an alternative to traditional open instrumentation and fusion, including the ability to stabilize patients with minimal blood loss and improved postoperative pain. Furthermore, improved trunk strength has been attributed to decreased soft tissue stripping.[8–12] Other studies have suggested that minimal violation and evacuation of the fracture hematoma is associated with local preservation of beneficial local cytokines and healing factors.[13,14] Other studies have shown similar fusion and functional outcomes as compared with open techniques.[8–10] Furthermore, fusionless techniques have been associated with preserved motion and improved functional outcomes. However, few data exist demonstrating this in the pediatric population.

A retrospective case series performed by Cui and colleagues[6] at a level 1 pediatric trauma center examined the outcomes of 14 patients treated with temporary PPSI for thoracic and lumbar fractures. Patients ranged in age from 10 to 18 years with comorbid injuries ranging from isolated trauma (8 patients) to polytrauma, including pelvis, extremity, chest, abdominal, and intracranial injuries. Spinal injuries in these patients included 4 patients with single-level injury and 10 patients with a multilevel injury. All were treated with percutaneous pedicle screws without fusion. Patients were selected based on difficult-to-brace segments (consecutive proximal thoracic fractures), concurrent

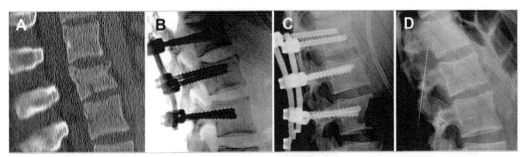

Fig. 1. Case 1. (A) A 17-year-old girl with an L2 burst fracture sustained in a motor vehicle collision. (B) An indirect reduction was accomplished through positioning and intraoperative screw-rod contouring and ligamentotaxis. (C) Maintenance of reduction is seen postoperatively and (D) 2 months after the removal of instrumentation. (From Cui S, Busel GA, Puryear AS. Temporary Percutaneous Pedicle Screw Stabilization Without Fusion of Adolescent Thoracolumbar Spine Fractures. J Pediatr Orthop 2016;36(7):701-8; with permission.)

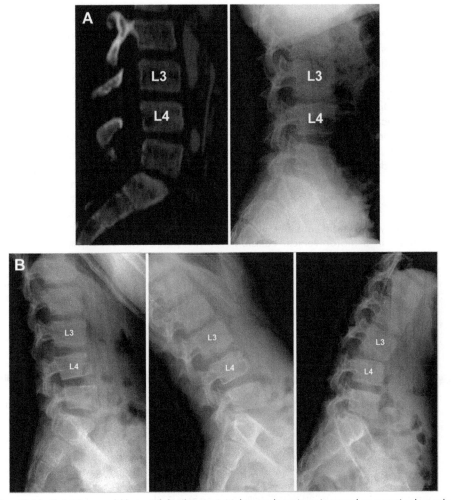

Fig. 2. Case 2. (A, B) A 12-year-old boy with back pain, initial recumbent imaging read as negative but subsequent spine clinic standing flexion/extension radiographs demonstrating L3-4 pure ligamentous chance injury. (From Cui S, Busel GA, Puryear AS. Temporary Percutaneous Pedicle Screw Stabilization Without Fusion of Adolescent Thoracolumbar Spine Fractures. J Pediatr Orthop 2016;36(7):701-8; with permission.)

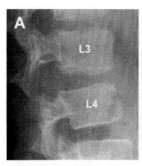
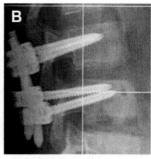
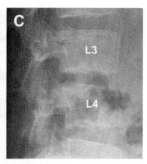

Fig. 3. Case 2. (*A*) L3-4 ligamentous chance injury (*B*) treated with short-segment percutaneous pedicle instrumentation. (*C*) Correction is maintained 30 months after the removal of instrumentation. (*From* Cui S, Busel GA, Puryear AS. Temporary Percutaneous Pedicle Screw Stabilization Without Fusion of Adolescent Thoracolumbar Spine Fractures. J Pediatr Orthop 2016;36(7):701-8; with permission.)

chest injury, or significant psychiatric disorders with increased risk of noncompliance or nontolerance with bracing.

All patients healed with significant improvements in radiographic parameters comparing pre/postsurgery. Duration of instrumentation was 5 to 12 months for 12 of the patients, with the remaining 2 initially lost to follow-up re-presenting 14 months and 32 months postoperatively due to symptomatic instrumentation desiring removal. Only 1 patient required subsequent surgery because of superficial wound dehiscence. No patients required further surgery to promote healing. At the latest follow-up, 93% of patients returned to preinjury activity levels.

Cases
Case 1
The patient is a 17-year old girl with an L2 burst fracture sustained in a motor vehicle collision

(**Fig. 1**). The patient was taken to the operating room for L1-L3 PPSI. An indirect reduction was accomplished through patient positioning and screw-rod contouring with ligamentotaxis. The patient healed with maintained alignment and position of instrumentation on follow-up radiographs. The patient subsequently underwent removal of instrumentation, and at 2 months, after removal demonstrated appropriate healing with maintained alignment.

Case 2
The patient is a 12-year old boy who presented with back pain following motor vehicle collision (**Fig. 2**A, B). Initial recumbent imaging taken on the initial trauma survey missed a ligamentous chance injury. The patient was treated initially with bracing. The patient subsequently presented to the pediatric orthopedic spine clinic with persistent back pain. Standing lateral

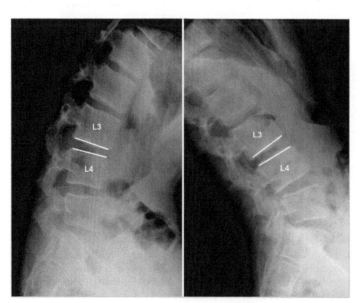

Fig. 4. Case 2. Radiographs taken 30 months after the removal of instrumentation demonstrates maintenance of arc of motion through the previously injured segment. (*From* Cui S, Busel GA, Puryear AS. Temporary Percutaneous Pedicle Screw Stabilization Without Fusion of Adolescent Thoracolumbar Spine Fractures. J Pediatr Orthop 2016;36(7):701-8; with permission.)

flexion/extension radiographs demonstrated a purely ligamentous chance injury, and the patient was later taken to the operating room for L3-L4 PPSI (**Fig. 3**). The patient underwent subsequent removal of instrumentation, and 30-month postoperative radiographs demonstrated maintained arc of motion through the injured segment without evidence of instability, posterior widening, or listhesis (**Fig. 4**).

SUMMARY

PPSI, with subsequent removal of instrumentation, is an attractive option for the management of pediatric spinal fractures. Although bracing remains the standard of care for most pediatric patients with spine trauma, PPSI offers significant advantages when bracing or casting may not be ideal or is otherwise contraindicated. Further studies, including additional prospective and multicenter research, are needed to better understand the role and broader clinical utility of this approach. However, existing studies and clinical experience so far suggest that temporary percutaneous fixation is a reasonable method of stabilization that guarantees compliance and promotes success in the management of select thoracic and lumbar spine fractures in the pediatric trauma patient.

DISCLOSURE

The authors have nothing to disclose.

REFERENCES

1. Akbarnia BA. Pediatric spine fractures. Orthop Clin North Am 1999;30:521–36, x.
2. Dogan S, Safavi-Abbasi S, Theodore N, et al. Thoracolumbar and sacral spinal injuries in children and adolescents: a review of 89 cases. J Neurosurg 2007;106:426–33.
3. Laer LV. Corrective mechanisms in the growing skeleton. In: von Laer L, editor. Pediatric fractures and dislocations. New York: Thieme; 2004. p. 11–8.
4. Karlsson MK, Moller A, Hasserius R, et al. A modeling capacity of vertebral fractures exists during growth: an up-to-47-year follow-up. Spine 2003;28:2087–92.
5. Moller A, Hasserius R, Besjakov J, et al. Vertebral fractures in late adolescence: a 27 to 47-year follow-up. Eur Spine J 2006;15:1247–54.
6. Cui S, Busel GA, Puryear AS. Temporary percutaneous pedicle screw stabilization without fusion of adolescent thoracolumbar spine fractures. J Pediatr Orthop 2016;36(7):701–8.
7. Cox JB, Yang M, Jacob RP, et al. Temporary percutaneous pedicle screw fixation for treatment of thoracolumbar injuries in young adults. J Neurol Surg A Cent Eur Neurosurg 2013;74:7–11.
8. Wang HW, Li CQ, Zhou Y, et al. Percutaneous pedicle screw fixation through the pedicle of fractured vertebra in the treatment of type A thoracolumbar fractures using Sextant system: an analysis of 38 cases. Chin J Traumatol 2010;13:137–45.
9. Wild MH, Glees M, Plieschnegger C, et al. Five-year follow-up examination after purely minimally invasive posterior stabilization of thoracolumbar fractures: a comparison of minimally invasive percutaneously and conventionally open treated patients. Arch Orthop Trauma Surg 2007;127:335–43.
10. Yang WE, Ng ZX, Koh KM, et al. Percutaneous pedicle screw fixation for thoracolumbar burst fracture: a Singapore experience. Singapore Med J 2012;53:577–81.
11. Kim DY, Lee SH, Chung SK, et al. Comparison of multifidus muscle atrophy and trunk extension muscle strength: percutaneous versus open pedicle screw fixation. Spine 2005;30:123–9.
12. Weber BR, Grob D, Dvorak J, et al. Posterior surgical approach to the lumbar spine and its effect on the multifidus muscle. Spine 1997;22:1765–72.
13. Grundnes O, Reikeras O. The importance of the hematoma for fracture healing in rats. Acta Orthop Scand 1993;64:340–2.
14. Ozaki A, Tsunoda M, Kinoshita S, et al. Role of fracture hematoma and periosteum during fracture healing in rats: interaction of fracture hematoma and the periosteum in the initial step of the healing process. J Orthop Sci 2000;5:64–70.

Percutaneous Osteotomies in Pediatric Deformity Correction

Nickolas Nahm, MD[a], Louise Reid Boyce Nichols, MD[b],*

KEYWORDS

- Percutaneous osteotomy • Corticotomy • Multiple drill hole osteotomy • Gigli saw osteotomy
- Focal dome osteotomy • Lower extremity deformity

KEY POINTS

- Percutaneous osteotomies decrease soft tissue injury and offer a low-energy method of cutting the bone to address lower extremity deformities.
- Types of percutaneous osteotomies include multiple drill hole osteotomy, corticotomy, and Gigli saw osteotomy.
- Deciding on the type of osteotomy to perform should take into account the anatomic location of the osteotomy and the necessary precision of the cut, with Gigli saw osteotomies offering the finest cut.

INTRODUCTION

Pediatric deformity correction frequently relies on the ability of bone to regenerate after an osteotomy rather than bone grafting.[1] The optimal osteotomy technique achieves this goal by minimizing injury to the bone and surrounding soft tissues and preserving the ability of bone to regenerate. Percutaneous osteotomy techniques are the best tools surgeons have to reduce injury to the soft tissue structures surrounding the bony osteotomy site.[2] Undertaking a minimally invasive approach also reduces damage to the vulnerable periosteal tissue and minimizes vascular disruption to the bone.[3] To decrease injury, the periosteum should be incised longitudinally (not transversely) and closed whenever possible after the osteotomy is completed.

Percutaneous osteotomies use instruments that are friendly to the bony structures and minimize heat generation.[4] Using a saw to cut bone through a larger open approach increases the risk of thermal necrosis, which is associated with poor bony healing.[5] Risk of thermal necrosis with a saw may be decreased by using a start-stop technique or by cooling the blade with cold normal saline fluid. Although percutaneous techniques are friendlier to the periosteum and soft tissue, they require a higher level of understanding of three-dimensional anatomy and are more technically demanding.

Percutaneous osteotomy techniques include the corticotomy,[3] multiple drill hole osteotomy,[1,2,6] and Gigli saw osteotomy.[1,2,7] All of these techniques use minimally invasive approaches. The corticotomy and multiple drill hole osteotomies produce the least heat. However, the corticotomy is less precise than the other techniques because it relies on rotational osteoclasis to complete the bone cut. This maneuver may result in an unpredictable bone cut and is not ideal for small structures, such as the bony structures in the foot. The Gigli saw osteotomy produces the cleanest and most accurate cut and may be most useful in areas with smaller

[a] International Center for Limb Lengthening, Rubin Institute for Advanced Orthopaedics, Sinai Hospital of Baltimore, 2401 West Belvedere Avenue, Baltimore, MD 21215, USA; [b] Department of Orthopaedic Surgery, Nemours AI duPont Hospital for Children, 1600 Rockland Avenue, Wilmington, DE 19803, USA
* Corresponding author.
E-mail address: reid.nichols@nemours.org

Orthop Clin N Am 51 (2020) 345–360
https://doi.org/10.1016/j.ocl.2020.03.001

anatomy.[8] However, the regenerate after Gigli saw osteotomy may be less robust than the regenerate after multiple drill hole osteotomy, and performance of this osteotomy is the most technically demanding.[9] The multiple drill hole osteotomy is most commonly performed and has reliable healing capacity. This article discusses percutaneous osteotomy techniques available in lower extremity pediatric deformity.

SURGICAL TECHNIQUES
Multiple Drill Hole Osteotomy

This technique may be applied to several different anatomic sites and is useful for creating transverse osteotomies and focal dome osteotomies.[3] The multiple drill hole osteotomy does not require rotational osteoclasis and may be useful in situations where a controlled osteotomy is required, such as when osteotomy needs to be performed adjacent to a half pin. This description focuses on application of the transverse osteotomy technique to the femoral shaft (Fig. 1) and the supracondylar region of the femur (Fig. 2). In addition, the multiple drill hole technique is used for creating focal dome osteotomies (Fig. 3) and is also useful in the proximal tibia (eg, correction of tibia vara) and the distal tibia (eg, derotational osteotomies).

After exposing the femur with a small incision, drilling is performed from lateral to medial (see Fig. 1). Care must be taken to avoid plunging past the medial cortex secondary to the location of the femoral artery. The size of the drill bit depends on the size of the bone. The drill is then withdrawn to the center of the bone and redirected anteromedially and posteromedially. An osteotome is then placed into the drill hole and directed with the same trajectory used by the drill bit. The trajectory should be verified with fluoroscopy. The osteotomy is completed by twisting the osteotome. A similar approach is used in the supracondylar region of the femur (see Fig. 2).

The focal dome osteotomy is a type of multiple drill hole osteotomy and is most frequently used in the distal femur and distal tibia. The main advantage of the focal dome osteotomy is improved bony contact. However, this technique is more technically demanding than other types of multiple drill hole osteotomies. In performing a focal dome osteotomy, the pivot point of the osteotomy is at the location of the center of rotation of angulation (CORA) of the deformity (see Fig. 3). A focal dome guide is required for the osteotomy and facilitates precise placement of the drill holes in an arc pattern. The distal tibia is exposed with a longitudinal

incision, and the focal dome guide is placed at the CORA. The surgeon drills multiple drill holes following the radius of curvature of the guide. Fibular osteotomy is performed through a separate small incision distal to the level of the tibial focal dome osteotomy. Guide pins for screw fixation are placed before completion of the osteotomy, and multiple osteotomes are used to complete the osteotomy.

To perform a multiple drill hole osteotomy of the tibia, drilling is performed first from anterior to posterior. The drill bit is then withdrawn to the center of the bone and redirected posteromedially and posterolaterally through the far cortex, being aware of the 3 neurovascular structures. Similar to the femur, an osteotome is used to complete the osteotomy. The osteotome is first directed anterior to posterior and then posteromedially and posterolaterally. The osteotome is then twisted 90° in order to complete the osteotomy.

Corticotomy

The first use of the corticotomy is generally attributed to Gavriil Ilizarov.[10] Through animal studies, Ilizarov found that preservation of endosteal tissues and blood supply improved bone regeneration. The goal of the corticotomy is to preserve the endosteal tissue by disrupting only the cortex with the osteotome followed by rotational osteoclasis for completion.[11,12] A corticotomy may be used in triangular (tibia, ulna, radius) and round (femur and humerus) bones.[1] In the tibia, a 5-mm to 10-mm incision is made over the crest of the tibia at the level of the osteotomy. An elevator is used to lift the periosteum from bone. Importantly, the lateral border of the tibia is straight from the anterior to posterior direction, whereas the medial surface is oblique. A 6.4-mm (0.25-inch) osteotome is used to cut the anterior half of the lateral cortex of the tibia up to the intramedullary canal. This distance is approximately 1 cm in adults, but cortical pitch may be used to guide the position of the osteotome. The cortical pitch represents the sound of the hammering of the osteotome when the osteotome is in cortical bone. The medial periosteum is then elevated, and the medial cortex is cut using the elevator as protection. Again, the cortical pitch may be used for guiding the osteotomy. The periosteal elevator may be palpated through the subcutaneous tissue to estimate the depth. Osteotomy of the lateral cortex is then completed with the elevator in place for protection. The elevator may be used to guide the trajectory of the osteotomy. An osteotome is placed in the lateral

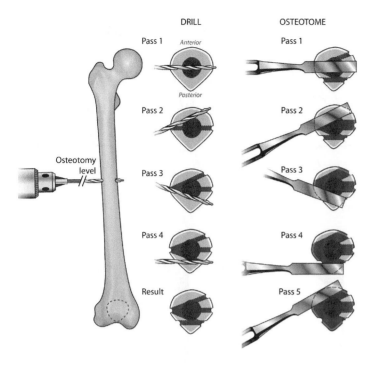

Fig. 1. Multiple drill hole osteotomy of the femoral shaft. Drill holes are made from lateral to medial, withdrawn to the center of the femoral shaft, and passed anteromedially and posteromedially. The osteotomy is completed with an osteotome. (© 2018 Rubin Institute for Advanced Orthopedics, Sinai Hospital of Baltimore, (Herzenberg JE, editor. The Art of Limb Alignment: Taylor Spatial Frame. 1st ed. Baltimore: Sinai Hospital of Baltimore, 2018.))

cortex and twisted. This maneuver spreads open the osteotomy site and opens the lateral cortex. The twisting maneuver with the osteotome is repeated on the medial cortex. An audible crack should be heard both medially and laterally before proceeding with osteoclasis. The osteotomy is completed with osteoclasis of the tibia. A rotational force is applied to the tibia to separate the fragments. In the proximal tibia, the distal fragment is rotated externally to avoid stretch injury to the peroneal nerve. This method may also be used in other triangular bones.

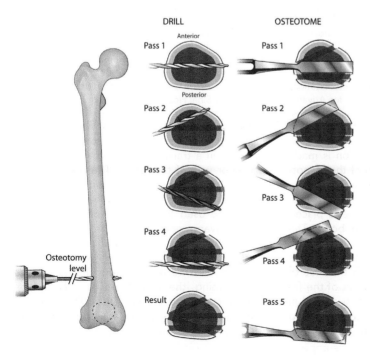

Fig. 2. Multiple drill hole osteotomy of the distal femur. In the supracondylar region of the femur, the bone is drilled from lateral to medial. The drill is withdrawn and aimed anteromedially and posteromedially. The osteotomy is completed with an osteotome. (© 2018 Rubin Institute for Advanced Orthopedics, Sinai Hospital of Baltimore, (Herzenberg JE, editor. The Art of Limb Alignment: Taylor Spatial Frame. 1st ed. Baltimore: Sinai Hospital of Baltimore, 2018.))

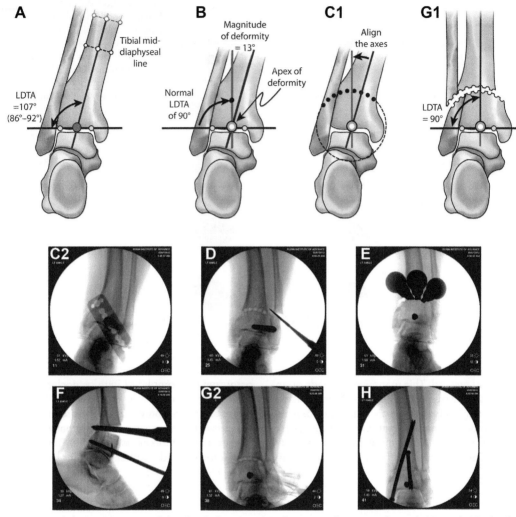

Fig. 3. Focal dome osteotomy of the distal tibia. (*A, B*) Deformity analysis is performed. (*C1* and *C2*) The focal dome guide facilitates placement of drill holes in an arm pattern. (*D*) Multiple drill hole osteotomy is made through the guide, and the fibular osteotomy is performed with an osteotome. (*E, F*) Multiple osteotomes are used to complete the focal dome osteotomy. (*G1* and *G2*) Proximal and distal tibial axes are aligned. (*H*) Before completion of the osteotomy, guidewires are placed for stabilization, and cannulated screws are placed for fixation. LDTA, lateral distal tibial angle. (© 2018 Rubin Institute for Advanced Orthopedics, Sinai Hospital of Baltimore.)

A corticotomy may also be used for round bones, including the femur and humerus.[3] For the femur, a 5-mm to 10-mm incision is made over the lateral thigh at the level of the osteotomy, and blunt dissection is carried down through subcutaneous tissue, fascia, and muscle. A 6.4-mm (0.25-inch) osteotome is placed in a longitudinal fashion down to bone. The osteotome is tapped against the bone and twisted 90°. Twisting the osteotome spreads the periosteum. The osteotome is then hit to create a groove on the lateral aspect of the femur. The osteotome is removed and angled in an anterolateral direction, with care to keep the osteotome in the corner of the groove.

These steps are performed for the posterolateral cortex as well. The osteotome should be oriented in a transverse fashion, parallel to the posterior wall of the femur. The posterior wall of the femur is the thickest part of the femur because of the linea aspera. The cortical pitch should be used to guide the depth of osteotome advancement. Once the cortical pitch changes, the osteotome is out of the posteromedial cortex of the bone. A wrench or vice grip can then be used to turn the osteotome 90°. Turning the osteotome in this fashion should crack the femur. Once this crack is achieved, rotational osteoclasis is used to complete the osteotomy.

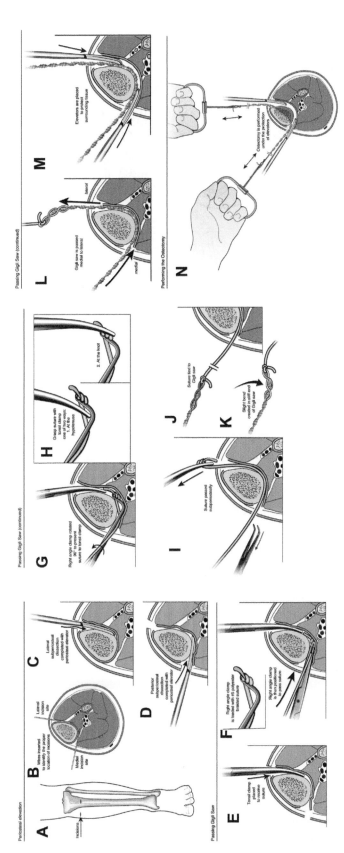

Fig. 4. Gigli saw osteotomy of the proximal tibia. (A) Two transverse incisions are placed (B) with wires used as guides. Subperiosteal dissection is performed with periosteal elevator (C) laterally and (D) medially. (E) Tonsil clamp is placed laterally to receive the suture. (F) A right-angle clamp is loaded with suture and placed in subperiosteal location medially. (G) Right-angle clamp is rotated to deliver suture around the posterolateral corner, and (H) suture is grasped with the tonsil clamp. (I) After suture passage, (J) the Gigli saw is tied to the suture on the medial side. (K) A bend is placed at the end of the Gigli saw to facilitate passage around the posterolateral corner. (L) The Gigli saw is passed, and (M) elevators are placed subperiosteally to protect the soft tissue. (N) Osteotomy is initiated. (O) Before completion of the osteotomy through the medial cortex, subperiosteal dissection of the medial cortex is performed with an elevator. Before exiting the medial cortex, (P) Senn retractors are placed to protect the skin. (Q) A palpable click designates completion of the osteotomy. Efforts should be made to preserve the medial periosteum. ([A–N] © 2013 Rubin Institute for Advanced Orthopedics, Sinai Hospital of Baltimore; and [O–Q] © 2019 Rubin Institute for Advanced Orthopedics, Sinai Hospital of Baltimore.)

Performing the Osteotomy (continued)

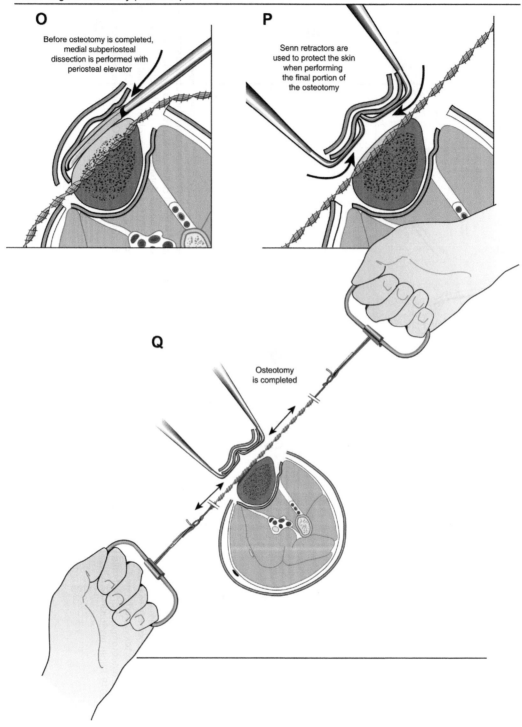

O Before osteotomy is completed, medial subperiosteal dissection is performed with periosteal elevator

P Senn retractors are used to protect the skin when performing the final portion of the osteotomy

Q Osteotomy is completed

Fig. 4. *(continued)*

Gigli Saw Osteotomy

Gigli saw osteotomy is used in the tibia, midfoot, and, less commonly, the femur. The Gigli saw should not be used in areas with thick diaphyseal cortical bone, because the saw may cause excessive heat generation and delay or prevent union. The osteotomy is performed with reciprocal back-and-forth motion of the Gigli saw, ensuring

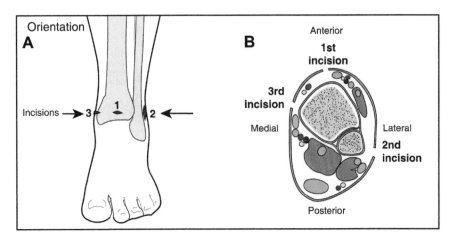

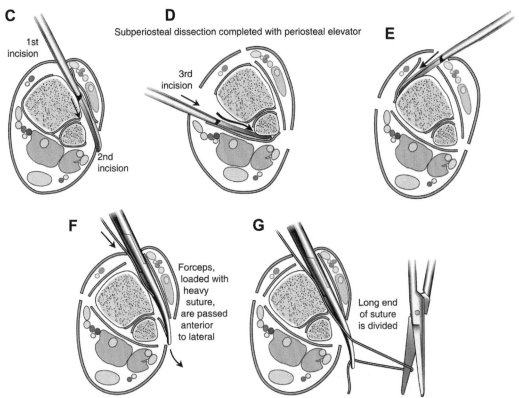

Fig. 5. Supramalleolar osteotomy with Gigli saw. (A, B) Two transverse incisions of the tibia and 1 longitudinal incision of the fibula are made. Subperiosteal dissection is performed (C) laterally, (D) posteriorly, and (E) medially with a periosteal elevator. (F, G) Suture is passed with long curved forceps from the anteromedial incision to the fibular incision and cut. (H) Forceps are removed, and (I) suture tied to the Gigli saw, which is (J) passed from the anteromedial incision to the fibular incision. (K and L) A second suture is passed from the posteromedial incision to the fibular incision and cut. (M, N) The forceps are removed, and the Gigli saw end at the fibular incision is tied to the suture. (O) The Gigli saw is passed, being careful to avoid kinking on the lateral side. (P) The bone is cut with reciprocal movement of the saw. (Q) Before completing the cut medially, an osteotome is placed to protect the medial structures. (R) The osteotomy is completed and (S) the saw removed. (© 2018 Rubin Institute for Advanced Orthopedics, Sinai Hospital of Baltimore, (Herzenberg JE, editor. The Art of Limb Alignment: Taylor Spatial Frame. 1st ed. Baltimore: Sinai Hospital of Baltimore, 2018.))

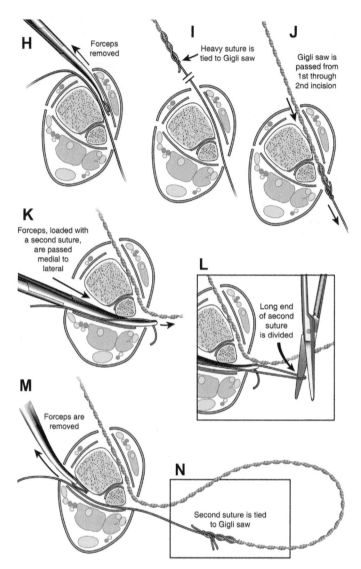

Fig. 5. (continued)

that the surrounding soft tissue is protected.[7] The advantage of the Gigli saw osteotomy compared with corticotomy is that rotational osteoclasis is not required, which is particularly useful when a bone defect is present, and when a precise cut is required in small structures, such as the midfoot.

The metaphyseal bone of the proximal tibia (Fig. 4) and distal tibia are ideal sites for Gigli saw osteotomy.[2] For the proximal tibia, 2 small separate transverse incisions (posteromedial and anterolateral) are made at the level of the osteotomy. The location of the incisions is guided by wire placement. Subperiosteal dissection of the tibia is performed with a periosteal elevator. A tonsil clamp is placed anterolaterally

to receive suture (eg, #5 polyester braided suture) placed at the posteromedial side. A right-angle clamp loaded with the suture is used to pass suture from posteromedial to anterolateral. Once in position to pass the suture, the right-angle clamp is rotated 90° to present the suture to the tonsil. The tonsil grasps the suture either at the knot or proximal to the knot. The tonsil should scrape along the bone as it is being passed. Whenever passing instruments, suture, or saw around the tibia, the toes should be observed. Flickering of the toes suggests irritation of the peroneal nerve.

The suture is tied to the Gigli saw, and a slight bend is placed at the end of the Gigli saw to ease passage around the posterolateral corner

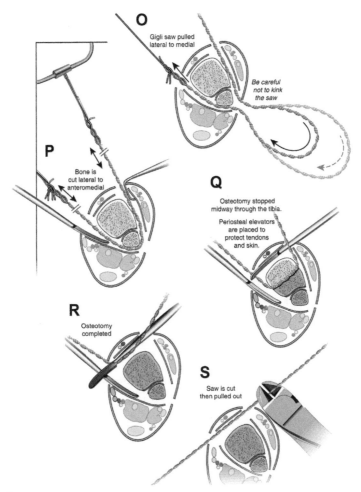

Fig. 5. (*continued*)

of the tibia. The Gigli saw is then passed from posterior to anterior using the suture. Elevators are placed subperiosteally on the medial and lateral sides to protect the soft tissues from the Gigli saw. In addition, elevators ensure that the Gigli saw is in a subperiosteal location. The osteotomy should be performed while the surgeon is standing on the medial side of the tibia to minimize skin issues. The 2 ends of the Gigli saw should be 90° to each other and should be moved in a reciprocal fashion. The posterior and lateral cortices of the tibia are cut with the Gigli saw under the protection of the elevators. After reaching the medial cortex, the angle of the Gigli saw is flattened, and an elevator is used to subperiosteally dissect the medial periosteum. Before the medial cut is finalized with the Gigli saw, 2 Senn retractors are placed to protect the skin. Cutting the medial cortex is the most difficult part. Grasping the wire with

the hands close together offers more control. A click may be palpated after exiting the medial cortex with the Gigli saw. Tensioning the saw may allow it to be palpated subcutaneously. Care should be taken to avoid cutting the medial periosteum. The saw is then cut and retrieved from the osteotomy site.

An inclined percutaneous Gigli saw osteotomy of the tibia is also possible.[1] A Kirschner wire is placed at the angle required for correction. Incisions are made at the proximal and distal ends of the wire. Subperiosteal elevation is performed laterally and medially. The elevation is anterior to posterior on the lateral side. On the medial side, the subperiosteal elevation is performed to meet the dissection performed on the lateral side. Suture is passed in a similar manner as was performed for the proximal tibia percutaneous osteotomy. Using a 90° clamp, suture is introduced subperiosteally on the medial

Orientation

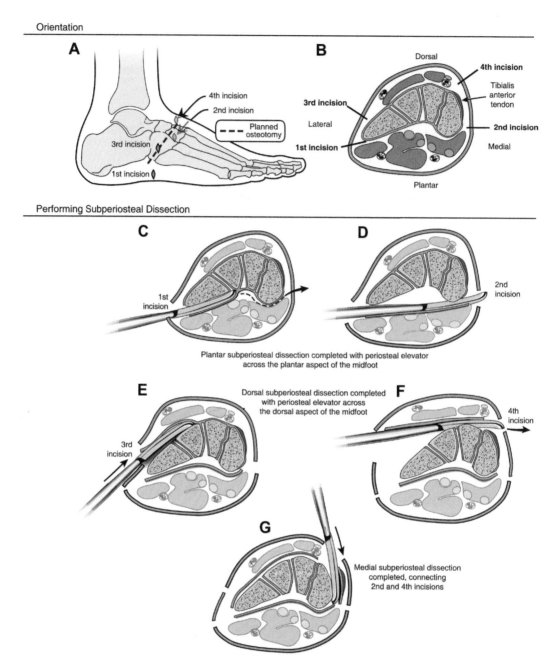

Performing Subperiosteal Dissection

Fig. 6. Midfoot osteotomy performed with Gigli saw. (*A, B*) Four incisions are used. Subperiosteal dissection is performed on the (*C, D*) plantar, (*E, F*) dorsal, and (*G*) medial surfaces. (*H, I*) Suture is passed from lateral to medial along the plantar surface. (*J, K*) Gigli saw is then passed along the plantar surface from medial to lateral. (*L, M*) Suture is then used to pass the Gigli saw along the medial surface. (*N–P*) The Gigli saw is bent to facilitate passage along the medial surface. (*Q–S*) In addition, the Gigli saw is passed along the dorsal surface. (*T*) The osteotomy is initiated and paused before completion along the lateral surface. (*U*) A periosteal elevator is placed under the lateral periosteum, and (*V*) the osteotomy is completed. (*W*) The Gigli saw is cut and removed. ([*A–M, T–W*] © 2011 Rubin Institute for Advanced Orthopedics, Sinai Hospital of Baltimore; and [*N–S*] © 2019 Rubin Institute for Advanced Orthopedics, Sinai Hospital of Baltimore.)

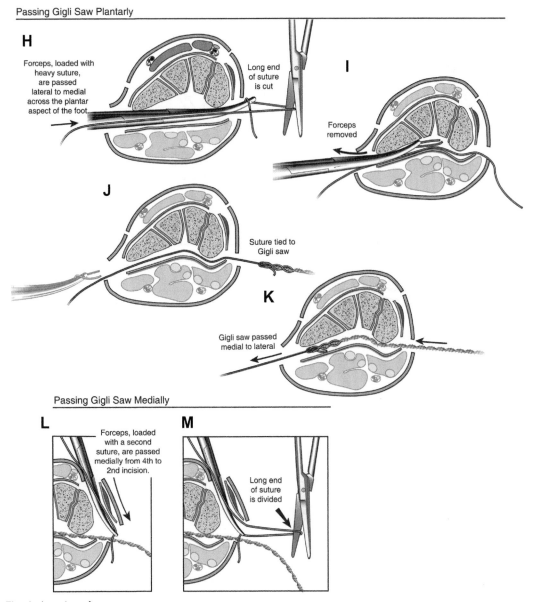

Passing Gigli Saw Plantarly

H Forceps, loaded with heavy suture, are passed lateral to medial across the plantar aspect of the foot.

Long end of suture is cut

I Forceps removed

J Suture tied to Gigli saw

K Gigli saw passed medial to lateral

Passing Gigli Saw Medially

L Forceps, loaded with a second suture, are passed medially from 4th to 2nd incision.

M Long end of suture is divided

Fig. 6. (*continued*)

side and retrieved with a long vascular clamp on the lateral side. The suture facilitates passage of the Gigli saw. The Gigli saw is placed distal to the Kirschner wire on the lateral side and proximal to the Kirschner wire on the medial side. The Kirschner wire is used to aid in performing the osteotomy. After reaching the medial cortex, the periosteum is elevated off the medial cortex along the path of the Kirschner wire after flattening the Gigli saw. The Gigli saw is then cut and removed. A similar approach is undertaken in the distal tibia with the Gigli saw passed around the tibia in a subperiosteal fashion from

anterior to posterior through 2 small transverse incisions. Elevators are used to protect the soft tissues, and the Gigli saw is used to cut the bone, similar to the proximal tibia.

In the supramalleolar region, no space exists between the tibia and the fibula, and both the tibia and the fibula are cut[13] (Fig. 5). For supramalleolar osteotomies, 3 small incisions are used: 2 transverse incisions over the medial tibia (anteromedial and posteromedial) and one longitudinal over the fibula.[2] Subperiosteal dissection is performed over the anterior tibia and anterior fibula. Placement of the fibular incision

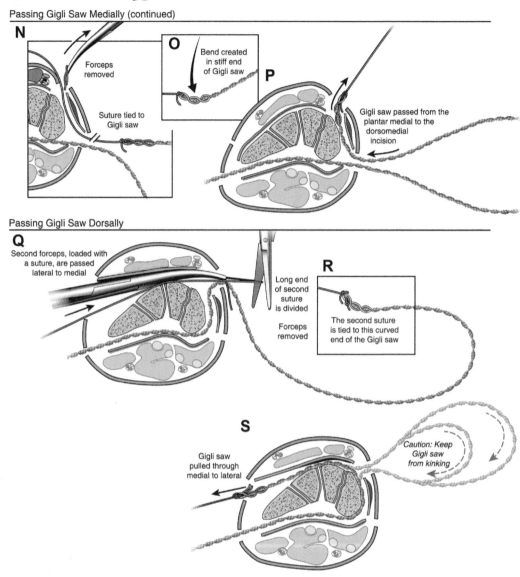

Fig. 6. (continued)

may be guided by placing an elevator from the anteromedial side and advanced over the fibula. A suture is passed from anteromedial to lateral with a long curved forceps. The suture is then tied to the Gigli saw, which is passed from anteromedial through the fibular incision. Subperiosteal dissection is performed on the posterior tibia and fibula through the posteromedial incision. A second suture is then passed from the posteromedial incision to fibular incision. The Gigli saw is then tied to the Gigli saw and passed from the fibular incision to the posteromedial incision. The medial periosteum of the tibia is elevated, and an elevator used to protect the soft tissue envelope. The Gigli saw is then used to cut the fibula and the tibia from lateral to medial, being careful to avoid kinking the saw. After the cut is complete, the Gigli saw is cut and pulled.

Gigli saw osteotomies may be performed in the midfoot at 3 levels: the neck of the talus and calcaneus, the cuboid-navicular, and the cuboid-cuneiform.[14] The location of the osteotomy depends on the apex of the deformity. Midfoot osteotomies are used for correction of cavovarus foot deformities gradually with a

Performing the Osteotomy

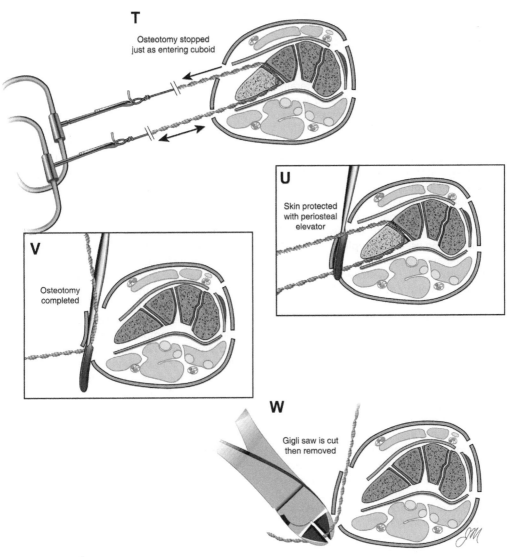

T

Osteotomy stopped
just as entering cuboid

U

Skin protected
with periosteal
elevator

V

Osteotomy
completed

W

Gigli saw is cut
then removed

Fig. 6. (continued)

frame. This approach is especially useful in young patients with small feet who cannot afford further shortening of the foot, which happens after wedge osteotomies performed for acute correction. Four small incisions (medial, lateral, dorsomedial, and dorsolateral) are made (**Fig. 6**). Subperiosteal dissection is performed through these incisions. Of note, subperiosteal elevation along the plantar surface may be difficult because of the concavity of the transverse arch. Using a mosquito clamp, the tips of the instrument should touch bone as the dissection is completed. Suture is used to facilitate passage of the Gigli saw from lateral to medial or medial to lateral. The Gigli saw is tied to the suture and passed plantar to the foot from a medial to lateral direction. The suture and saw are then passed through the dorsomedial incision using a long curved clamp. The Gigli saw is then passed in a subperiosteal fashion around the dorsum of the foot. Using periosteal elevators to protect the soft tissues, the Gigli saw is then used to cut the bone. The lateral periosteum is elevated and protected, and the cut is finished. The saw is then cut and removed.

In the distal femur, the multiple drill hole technique is more commonly used and easier to perform than Gigli saw osteotomy. However, a Gigli saw osteotomy may be faster to perform than the multiple drill hole technique. To perform a Gigli saw osteotomy of the distal femur, 2 small transverse incisions are made, 1 anteromedially and the other posterolaterally.[1] Two Kirschner wires may be placed to localize the borders of the femur. Subperiosteal dissection is performed posteriorly and medially. A right-angle clamp is used to pass suture and is retrieved on the medial side with a long curved clamp. Passage of the Gigli saw is facilitated by the suture. The Gigli saw is used to only cut the posterior and medial cortices. Cutting into the anterior cortex may damage the quadriceps muscle and tendon because of saw injury. An osteotome may be used to complete the osteotomy along the anterior cortex.

Percutaneous Gigli saw osteotomy in the proximal femur is also not commonly used. The multiple drill hole and osteotome technique is quicker and less traumatic compared with the Gigli saw. However, the use of a Gigli saw is most helpful in the proximal femur when an osteotomy needs to be performed around an intramedullary nail.[15] The Gigli saw can be used to cut the medial cortex, and osteotomy of the remaining cortices is completed with an osteotome. In order to introduce the Gigli saw, 2 lateral transverse incisions are made anterior and posterior to the femur. Two Kirschner wires may be used to localize the anterior and posterior borders of the femur. Subperiosteal dissection is performed from the lateral side both posteriorly and anteriorly. Suture is passed from posterior to anterior using a 90° clamp. The suture is retrieved with a long curved clamp. The surgeon must be certain that the dissection and instruments are subperiosteal in order to prevent damage to the nearby neurovascular structures. The Gigli saw is passed around the femur after tying to the suture. The femur is cut from medial to lateral with the Gigli saw until it reaches the intramedullary nail. The Gigli saw is cut and removed and the remaining cortices are cut with a narrow osteotome.

DISCUSSION

The advantages of percutaneous osteotomies include decreased soft tissue dissection, minimizing trauma to adjacent tissues, preserving the osseous blood supply, and optimizing the healing environment for the osteotomy.[1] However, performing percutaneous osteotomies is technically demanding. Risk of neurovascular injury as well as incomplete osteotomy is theoretically higher with percutaneous approaches. Adequate subperiosteal dissection is crucial to avoid neurovascular injury. Maintaining subperiosteal position with passing of all instruments, suture, and Gigli saw is also vital. Furthermore, performance of these osteotomies requires a strong awareness of the three-dimensional anatomy of the structure of interest. In addition, tactile and auditory feedback from the instruments is a critical part of performing the osteotomies and helps in the safe and successful completion of the osteotomy. Performance of percutaneous osteotomies with an experienced partner or mentor may ease the learning curve for the operator and decrease risk for the patient when first performing these techniques.

Previous studies comparing percutaneous osteotomy techniques do not clearly favor one technique rather than the other. In 1 study examining tibial lengthening without deformity correction, Eralp and colleagues[16] found that Gigli saw osteotomy was associated with better healing index compared with multiple drill hole osteotomy. Another study comparing multiple drill hole osteotomy with Gigli saw osteotomy found that multiple drill hole osteotomy was associated with incomplete osteotomy as well as bone fracture.[17] Interestingly, this study found a lower healing index for the Gigli saw osteotomy compared with the multiple drill hole osteotomy, which may be related to increased heat generation compared with multiple drill hole osteotomies. Further prospective, randomized clinical trials are required to determine the efficacy of each technique.

The senior author prefers the Gigli saw osteotomy in tibia vara cases using gradual correction. The Gigli saw allows for a high tibial osteotomy in metaphyseal bone close to the apex of the deformity when using a hexapod fixator and gradual correction. The correction of cavovarus foot with midfoot osteotomy or low supramalleolar osteotomy with hexapod fixator are also common scenarios for this technique (Figs. 7 and 8). The Gigli saw osteotomy affords an accurate cut, especially in the midfoot, with minimal bone loss. Multiple drill hole osteotomy is useful in the femur, because passing the Gigli saw may be difficult and may put neurovascular structures at risk. Multiple drill hole osteotomy may be considered in patients requiring a diaphyseal osteotomy or dome osteotomy, which increases bony contact for healing.

To conclude, this article provides an overview of percutaneous osteotomy techniques in

A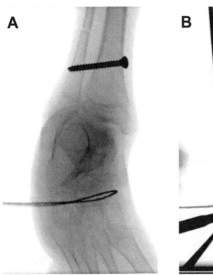

B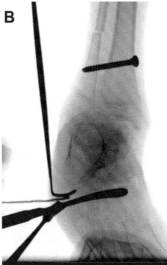

Fig. 7. (*A, B*) Midfoot osteotomy with Gigli saw.

pediatric lower extremity deformity. The main categories of percutaneous osteotomies include the Ilizarov corticotomy, multiple drill hole osteotomy, and Gigli saw osteotomy. Each technique has distinct advantages and disadvantages and requires a certain level of experience to perform safely and effectively. Nevertheless, percutaneous osteotomies, in terms of minimizing soft tissue injury and maximizing healing potential, have high potential benefit to the patients.

DISCLOSURE

The authors have nothing to disclose.

REFERENCES

1. Paley D. Principles of deformity correction. Berlin: Springer; 2002.
2. Herzenberg J. The art of limb alignment: taylor spatial frame. Baltimore, MD: Rubin Institute for Advanced Orthopedics, Sinai Hospital of Baltimore; 2018.
3. Paley D, Tetsworth K. Percutaneous osteotomies. Osteotome and Gigli saw techniques. Orthop Clin North Am 1991;22(4):613–24.
4. Dabis J, Templeton-Ward O, Lacey AE, et al. The history, evolution and basic science of osteotomy techniques. Strategies Trauma Limb Reconstr 2017;12(3):169–80.
5. Frierson M, Ibrahim K, Boles M, et al. Distraction osteogenesis. A comparison of corticotomy techniques. Clin Orthop 1994;(301):19–24.
6. Yasui N, Nakase T, Kawabata H, et al. A technique of percutaneous multidrilling osteotomy for limb lengthening and deformity correction. J Orthop Sci 2000;5(2):104–7.
7. Wardak MM, Wardak E. Percutaneous Gigli saw osteotomy. Oper Orthop Traumatol 2010;22(4): 414–20.

Fig. 8. Supramalleolar osteotomy with Gigli saw.

8. Tomita K, Kawahara N. The threadwire saw: a new device for cutting bone. J Bone Joint Surg Am 1996;78(12):1915–7.

9. Catagni MA, Guerreschi F, Lovisetti L. Distraction osteogenesis for bone repair in the 21st century: lessons learned. Injury 2011;42(6):580–6.

10. Aronson J. Limb-lengthening, skeletal reconstruction, and bone transport with the Ilizarov method. J Bone Joint Surg Am 1997;79(8):1243–58.

11. Hosny GA, Ahmed A-SA-A, Hussein MA-E. Clinical outcomes with the corticotomy-first technique associated with the Ilizarov method for the management of the septic long bones non-union. Int Orthop 2018;42(12):2933–9.

12. De Bastiani G, Aldegheri R, Renzi-Brivio L, et al. Limb lengthening by callus distraction (callotasis). J Pediatr Orthop 1987;7(2):129–34.

13. Eidelman M, Katzman A, Zaidman M, et al. Deformity correction using supramalleolar gigli saw osteotomy and Taylor spatial frame: how to perform this osteotomy safely? J Pediatr Orthop B 2011;20(5):318–22.

14. Eidelman M, Keren Y, Katzman A. Correction of residual clubfoot deformities in older children using the Taylor spatial butt frame and midfoot Gigli saw osteotomy. J Pediatr Orthop 2012;32(5):527–33.

15. Azzam W, El-Sayed M. Ilizarov distraction osteogenesis over the preexisting nail for treatment of nonunited femurs with significant shortening. Eur J Orthop Surg Traumatol 2016;26(3):319–28.

16. Eralp L, Kocaoğlu M, Ozkan K, et al. A comparison of two osteotomy techniques for tibial lengthening. Arch Orthop Trauma Surg 2004;124(5):298–300.

17. Makhdoom A, Kumar J, Siddiqui AA. Ilizarov external fixation: percutaneous gigli saw versus multiple drill-hole osteotomy techniques for distraction osteogenesis. Cureus 2019;11(6):e4973.

Hand and Wrist

Endoscopic Carpal Tunnel Release
Indications, Technique, and Outcomes

Efstathios Karamanos, MD[a], Bao-Quynh Jillian, MD[a],
David Person, MD[b],*

KEYWORDS

- Carpal tunnel • Endoscopic release • Technique • Outcomes

KEY POINTS

- Carpal tunnel is the most common peripheral compressive neuropathy.
- Nonoperative management may provide temporary alleviation of symptoms, but in most cases, surgical decompression is warranted.
- There are a multitude of approaches ranging from open release under general anesthesia to wide awake in-office endoscopic carpal tunnel release.

INTRODUCTION

Carpal tunnel syndrome or median nerve neuropathy at the wrist is the most common compressive peripheral neuropathy in the general population, with a prevalence that is as high as 3.8%.[1] Carpal tunnel syndrome can result in significant disability, which can translate to a heavy economic burden with most patients recovering to only about half of their preinjury earnings compared with patients with upper extremity fractures.[2]

As a result, proper diagnosis and treatment are of paramount importance. Nonsurgical treatment can be offered to those patients who experience mild to moderate symptomatology. Steroid injections are the mainstay of conservative treatment, with demonstrated significant short-term benefits.[3] Other nonsurgical treatments, such as wearing a splint, the use of therapeutic ultrasound, or oral corticosteroids, have demonstrated little to no benefit in the treatment of carpal tunnel syndrome.[4]

Although conservative management leads to a temporary alleviation of symptoms, when the symptoms recur, a surgical approach is indicated. The surgery involves incising the transverse carpal ligament, which in turn results in alleviation of pressure and compression of the contents of the carpal tunnel, including the median nerve (Fig. 1). One of the most dreadful complications is injury to the neurovascular structures. Those include, but are not limited to, the ulnar neurovascular bundle in Guyon's canal, the superficial palmar arch and the recurrent motor branch of the median nerve. Although all of these factors can result in significant morbidity, an injury to the recurrent motor branch of the median nerve can result in significant loss of hand function and thumb opposition. Preservation of the nerve is of particular importance, given the anatomic variances that can be encountered during dissection of the wrist or division of the transverse carpal ligament[5–8] (see Fig. 1; Fig. 2).

In endoscopic carpal tunnel release (ECTR), the motor branch is usually excluded by the instrumentation in the author's experience. When visualized, it can easily be avoided, or conversion to an open procedure is considered if believed to be more judicious.

Although there is good evidence to support the superiority of surgical treatment in relieving symptoms compared with nonsurgical treatment[9]

---

[a] Division of Plastic and Reconstructive Surgery, Department of Surgery, UT Health San Antonio, 7703 Floyd Curl Drive, San Antonio, TX 78229, USA; [b] The Hand Center of San Antonio, 21 Spurs Lane # 310, San Antonio, TX 78240, USA
* Corresponding author.
E-mail address: davidpersonmd@gmail.com

0030-5898/20/© 2020 Elsevier Inc. All rights reserved.

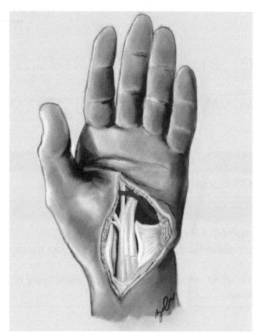

Fig. 1. Anatomy of the carpal tunnel. With the transverse carpal ligament incised, the most superficial (and radial) structure encountered is the median nerve. Notice the recurrent motor branch on the radial side of the nerve. Also note the proximity (reference) of the superficial palmar arch to the distal edge of the transverse carpal ligament. (*Illustrated by* B.Q. Julian, MD, San Antonio, TX.)

there is no consensus with regards to the surgical approach. Both open carpal tunnel release and ECTR are widely popular, with advocates for both approaches.[10] A Cochrane review by Vasiliadis and colleagues[11] concluded that both approaches are equally effective in improving functional status with a slight better improvement of grip strength in the ECTR group. The same group concluded that, although minor complications were lower in the ECTR group, major complications were no different. In contrast, a recent study by Michelotti and colleagues[12] by Penn State University failed to show any differences in the outcomes between patient that underwent an endoscopic and an open approach. However, they noted that patients preferred an endoscopic approach, demonstrated by their higher satisfaction scores.

Although the choice between endoscopic and open approach is still controversial, the endoscopic approach may improve strength in the early postoperative period,[13] but it is associated with a higher risk of nerve injury (neuropraxia) and depends on the surgeon's experience (Table 1). Furthermore, return to work is still controversial and is usually left in

the discretion of the surgeon. Little evidence exists regarding resuming unrestricted activities between endoscopic or open carpal tunnel release at 1 week postoperatively. The present article will be discussing the surgical technique of ECTR.

SURGICAL TECHNIQUE
Preoperative Planning

Carpal tunnel syndrome is a clinical syndrome and, as such, its diagnosis relies heavily on history and physical examination. One can further evaluate the patient with electromyography, if needed. A complete history, including previous open or endoscopic releases of the carpal tunnel, previous injuries to the hand, and other compression neuropathies should be obtained. An Allen test should be performed to assess the blood supply to the hand. It is also important to document a complete motor/sensory examination of the affected hand before ECTR. Any conditions (such as diabetic neuropathy) should be carefully documented. A full list of medication, including any supplements should be obtained. The patient should be advised that ECTR is performed in an outpatient setting. Bilateral ECTRs are feasible, but the patient should be advised that owing to injection of local anesthetic, hand dexterity may be impaired for the duration of action of the local anesthetic and, as such, support from a family member will be needed during that time.

There are 2 general approaches to ECTR: 2 incision (Chow technique) and 1 incision. The 2 incision is antiquated in the senior author's opinion and may add to injury to the common digital nerve to the third webspace and neuropraxia. Furthermore, some systems use direct in-line optics with no working port. Others use a 30° scope and have a working port to aid in tactile feedback to define the distal aspect of the ligament and rasping under direct visualization. Although there is no evidence to suggest the superiority of 1 versus 2 portal techniques in terms of outcomes, this article delineates the surgical approach using the single incision, antegrade approach to ECTR using the SEGWay system (SEGway Orthopaedics, Carlsbad, CA) and technique.

Patient Preparation and Positioning

The senior author's preference is to perform the procedure under general anesthesia, but use of local anesthesia with administration of intravenous sedation is routinely performed by the author, depending on the patient's anesthetic risk. Some surgeons perform this procedure in

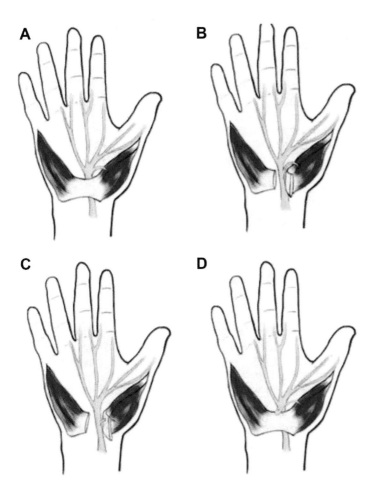

Fig. 2. Variations of the anatomy recurrent motor branch of the median nerve. (*A*) Extraligamentous. (*B*) Subligamentous. (*C*) Transligamentous. (*D*) Ulnar origin. (*Illustrated by* B.Q. Julian, MD, San Antonio, TX.)

Table 1	
Advantages and disadvantages of ECTR	
Advantages	**Disadvantages**
Small incisions	Higher incidence
Faster	of temporary
Avoids secondary	nerve injury
scarring of the	Expensive equipment
nerve	Steep learning curve
Allows concurrent	
bilateral	
treatment	
Better early grip	
strength	
Lower incidence	
of minor	
complications	
Higher patient	
satisfaction	
Better scar	
appearance	

the wide-awake patient. The airway is protected with a laryngeal mask airway. A nonsterile tourniquet is placed at the level the axilla of the upper extremity and the arm is draped in the usual fashion. If the surgeon is right-hand dominant, the position should be in such a way so that his or her right hand is facing the hand and the left hand is facing the forearm; if the procedure involves the left hand, the surgeon should be sitting toward the patient's head, and vice versa if the ECTR involves the left hand. The opposite positions should be assumed if the surgeon is left-hand dominant. The senior author prefers to place the endoscopy tower on the patient's left side, regardless of the laterality of the disease. The procedure is performed in the sitting position. The scrub tech is sitting opposite to the surgeon. If a bilateral procedure is to be performed, the senior author prefers both upper extremities to be prepped and draped before the beginning of the procedure (**Fig. 3**).

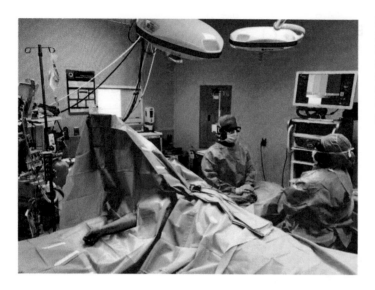

Fig. 3. Patient and surgeon setup. Notice that both hands are draped before the beginning of the procedure. The endoscopy tower is placed on the patient's left. The surgeon is about to perform an ECTR on the left hand and is sitting toward the patient's head.

Surgical Procedure
Incision

The palmaris longus tendon is identified (Fig. 4). If present, the skin incision should be made immediately ulnar to the palmaris longus tendon, about 1 to 2 cm proximal to the distal wrist crease. If there is no palmaris longus tendon, the incision should be centered between the radial border of the ring finger and Guyon's canal. The incision does not need to be longer than 1 cm (Fig. 5). For the sake of this discussion, we assume that the surgeon performing the procedure is right-hand dominant. Before incision the arm is elevated, a compression bandage is used to exsanguinate the extremity and the tourniquet is inflated to 250 mm Hg.

> *Step 1:* The skin is incised. Superficial veins will be encountered at this level. Using a hemostat, a gentle spread is performed superficially in the direction of the incision, which generally sweeps the veins out of the field. If the veins cannot be spread away from the incision, then they may be transected or cauterized with bipolar cautery.
>
> *Step 2:* Dissection is carried down to the antebrachial fascia. Once the antebrachial

```
┌─────────────────────────────────────┐
│          Incise the skin             │
└─────────────────────────────────────┘
                  ↓
┌─────────────────────────────────────┐
│     Incise the antebrachial fascia   │
└─────────────────────────────────────┘
                  ↓
┌─────────────────────────────────────┐
│  Enter the space above the median nerve │
└─────────────────────────────────────┘
                  ↓
┌─────────────────────────────────────┐
│   Scrape the undersurface of the TCL │
└─────────────────────────────────────┘
                  ↓
┌─────────────────────────────────────┐
│           Dilate the space           │
└─────────────────────────────────────┘
                  ↓
┌─────────────────────────────────────┐
│           Insert endoscope           │
└─────────────────────────────────────┘
                  ↓
┌─────────────────────────────────────────────┐
│ Use a rasp to clean the undersurface of the TCL │
└─────────────────────────────────────────────┘
                  ↓
┌─────────────────────────────────────┐
│  Use a probe to identify distal end of TCL │
└─────────────────────────────────────┘
                  ↓
┌─────────────────────────────────────┐
│     Cut TCL with endoscopic knife    │
└─────────────────────────────────────┘
                  ↓
┌─────────────────────────────────────┐
│  Inspect for complete transection of TCL │
└─────────────────────────────────────┘
                  ↓
┌─────────────────────────────────────┐
│   Incise proximal antebrachial fascia │
└─────────────────────────────────────┘
                  ↓
┌─────────────────────────────────────┐
│ Inject local anesthetic – close the incision │
└─────────────────────────────────────┘
```

Fig. 4. Step-by-step description of ECTR as performed by the senior author. TCL, transverse carpal ligament.

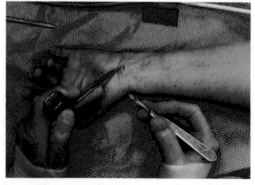

Fig. 5. Placement of incision.

fascia is encountered, it is grasped with a second hemostat. Using a 15 blade knife, the fascia is gently pressed with the belly of the knife to incise it. The edge of the now incised fascia is grabbed with the hemostat.

Step 3: With the remaining hemostat, the tissue is spread again in the direction of the incision until the space where the median nerve travels distally toward the carpal tunnel is visualized.

Comment: The identification of the correct space, as described, is one of the most critical parts of the procedure and successful identification depends on the surgeon's experience.

Step 4: With the surgeon's left hand supinated, the thumb is placed in the patient's palm at the distal end of the transverse carpal ligament between the hook of the hamate and the thenar eminence and gently press. The rest of the surgeon's fingers should be placed on the dorsal aspect of the patient's hand and wrist and gently press upwards to slightly extend it.

Comment: From now on, the surgeon's right arm remains adducted and touching the surgeon's torso at all times. This positioning provides maximal control of finger movements during the rest of the procedure and avoids gross motor movements of the arm to maximize safety and control (**Fig. 6**).

Step 5: The surgeon's right hand inserts a rasp to scrape the inflammatory synovium from the undersurface of the transverse carpal ligament. The surgeon's left thumb will feel the dilator through the carpal tunnel distal to the transverse carpal ligament. Tactile feedback from the transverse fibers of the transverse carpal ligament confirm adequate clearing of the synovium.

Step 6: Once complete, the surgeon passes successively increasing sized dilators into the space just created. One pass of each dilator should be adequate.

Comment: Once the endoscope is inserted, the surgeon stabilizes the guide (camera and working ports) using the left hand. The scrub tech drives the endoscope.

Step 7: At this point the endoscope is inserted. The rest of the procedure is done under endoscopic guidance a 30°, 4-mm scope (a smaller guide using a 2.7-mm scope is also available for smaller wrists). The view is explained in **Fig. 7**. The undersurface of the transverse carpal ligament is inspected under direct visualization. If there is need for further removal of synovium, that is, performed under direct visualization with the use of an endoscopic rasp (**Fig. 8**).

Step 8: A probe is then inserted and the distal end of the transverse carpal ligament is identified. This is done to avoid incomplete release of the transverse carpal ligament and avoid injury to more distal structures such as the palmar arch (**Fig. 9**).

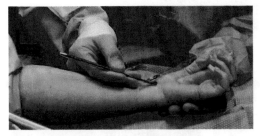

Fig. 6. Ergonomics of the procedure. The surgeon is dilating the space for the endoscope. Note the surgeon's hands; the left hand is supinated with the thumb gently pressing to feel for the distal end of the dilator while the rest of the fingers are supporting the patient's hand. The right arm is resting on the surgeon's side for stabilization while the hand is supinated. All surgical motions are performed using only the wrist and the fingers.

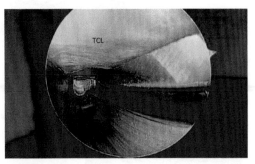

Fig. 7. Endoscopic view with the camera inserted. Note on the upper side of the view, the transverse carpal ligament (TCL). The median nerve is underneath and protected from any potential injury. Also note that the TCL has been cleaned from inflammatory synovium by using the rasp before inserting the endoscope.

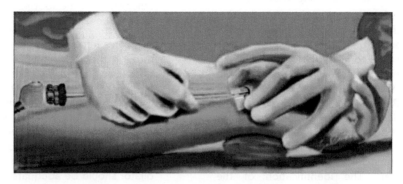

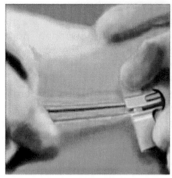
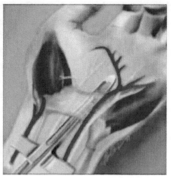
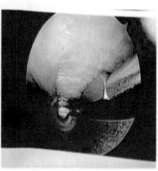

Fig. 8. An endoscopic rasp is inserted and any remaining synovium is removed. (*Illustrated by* B.Q. Julian, MD, San Antonio, TX.)

Step 9: The endoscopic knife is inserted under direct visualization. The transverse carpal ligament is divided (**Fig. 10**).

Step 10: Once the knife is removed, the transverse carpal ligament is inspected to ensure complete transection of the transverse carpal ligament. This is evidenced by wide, parallel separation of the leaflets, loss of tension on the leaflets and more proximal prolapsing fat.

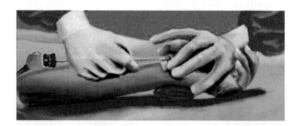

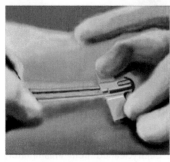
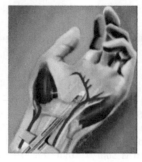
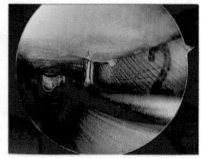

Fig. 9. Once the transverse carpal ligament is cleared from synovium, a probe is used to identify its distal edge under direct visualization. (*Illustrated by* B.Q. Julian, MD, San Antonio, TX.)

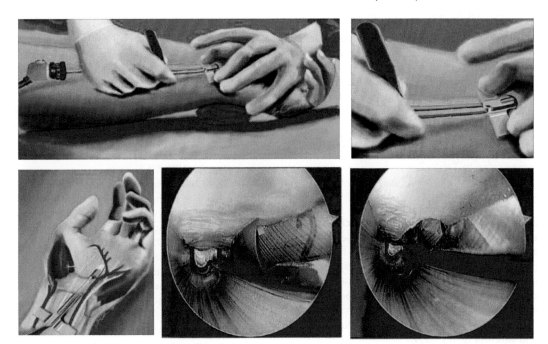

Fig. 10. The endoscopic knife is inserted and the transverse carpal ligament is divided. (*Illustrated by* B.Q. Julian, MD, San Antonio, TX.)

Table 2 Complications	
Complication	**Management**
Recurrence	Repeat ECRT Consider open carpal tunnel release Consider another etiology (eg, ganglion cyst)
Bleeding or hematoma	Observe, evacuate if compression develops
Infection	Elevation, antibiotics, incision and drainage if severe
Hypertrophic scar	Steroid injection, revision if pain is persistent
Reflex sympathetic dystrophy	Medical management
Scarring of the median nerve	Surgical release of the nerve
Injury to the recurrent motor branch	Nerve repair if possible
Injury to the flexor tendons	Surgical repair
Injury to the main median nerve	Surgical repair
Injury to the ulnar neurovascular bundle	Surgical repair

Step 11: Using Metzenbaum scissors, the antebrachial fascia is incised proximal to the incision for about 2 cm.

Step 12: Eight to 10 mL of 0.25% bupivicaine with epinephrine is injected around the incision and the palm at the operative site for postoperative analgesia and hemostasis. The tourniquet is released. The use of bipolar cautery is occasionally necessary. The skin is closed with a 4-0 nylon suture in a subcuticular fashion as a pull out suture. A sterile dressing is applied.

In-line systems are very similar in the overall approach to ECTR. In these systems, the blade and camera are incorporated in a single device. This combination allows direct visualization of the cut ligament (as opposed to a slightly offset cut). They do, however, lack the ability to rasp or probe under direct visualization (which are designed to enhance safety). For these systems, the steps as described are essentially the same, minus steps 7 and 8. Commonly used examples of these devices are MicroAire and Centerline (Arthrex, Naples, FL), discussed elsewhere in this article.

Postoperative Care

One of the major advantages of ECTR is the minimal down time from work and daily activities. At the conclusion of the procedure, a sterile soft dressing is applied at the site of the incision. We do not use a splint postoperatively, which in turn allows for early mobility and less development of postoperative stiffness. The dressing is removed at 24 hours and the patient is allowed to return to activities at 1 week. No antibiotics are prescribed. Narcotic pain medication is not routinely prescribed.

COMPLICATIONS AND MANAGEMENT

Please refer to Table 2.

SUMMARY

ECTR is a safe and effective approach to carpal tunnel release. It involves minimal down time and rapid return to work. Costs are higher, but this factor may be mitigated by the societal impact of earlier return to work. In-office procedures are becoming increasingly popular and some companies have developed in office systems that use some disposable instrumentation and wireless technology.

DISCLOSURE

DP is a minor shareholder in SEGWay Orthopedics, which is a division of Trice Medical. DWP is on the speaker's bureau for Trice Medical. The remaining authors have no relevant financial disclosures.

REFERENCES

1. Atroshi I, Gummesson C, Johnsson R, et al. Prevalence of carpal tunnel syndrome in a general population. JAMA 1999;282(2):153–8.
2. Foley M, Silverstein B, Polissar N. The economic burden of carpal tunnel syndrome: long-term earning of CTS claimants in Washington State. Am J Ind Med 2007;50(3):155–72.
3. Piazzini DB, Aprile I, Ferrara PE, et al. A systematic review of conservative treatment of carpal tunnel syndrome. Clin Rehabil 2007;21(4):299–314.
4. Page MJ, Massy-Westropp N, O'Connor D, et al. Splinting for carpal tunnel syndrome. Cochrane Database Syst Rev 2012;(7):CD010003.
5. Rotman MB, Donovan JP. Practical anatomy of the carpal tunnel. Hand Clin 2002;18(2):219–30.
6. Hong JT, Lee SW, Han SH, et al. Anatomy of neurovascular structures around the carpal tunnel during wrist motion for endoscopic carpal tunnel release. Neurosurgery 2006;58(1 Suppl):ONS127–33 [discussion: ONS127–33].
7. Al-Qattan MM. Variation in the course of the thenar motor branch of the median nerve and their relationship to the hypertrophic muscle overlying the transverse carpal ligament. J Hand Surg Am 2010; 35(11):1820–4.
8. Henry BM, Zwinczewska H, Roy J, et al. The prevalence of anatomic variations of the median nerve in the carpal tunnel: a systematic review and meta-analysis. PLoS One 2015;10(8): e0136477.
9. Verdugo RJ, Salinas RA, Castillo JL, et al. Surgical versus non-surgical treatment for carpal tunnel syndrome. Cochrane Database Syst Rev 2008;(4):CD001552.
10. Satteson ES, Cunningham TC, Gerard J, et al. Single surgeon series of outcomes of 897 consecutive endoscopic carpal tunnel releases stratified by disease severity. J Plast Reconstr Aesthet Surg 2019; 72(1):137–71.
11. Vasiliadis HS, Georgoulas P, Shrier I, et al. Endoscopic Release for carpal tunnel syndrome. Cochrane Database Syst Rev 2014;(1):CD008265.
12. Michelotti B, Romanowsky D, Hauck RM, et al. Prospective, randomized evaluation of endoscopic versus open carpal tunnel release in bilateral carpal tunnel syndrome: an interim analysis. Ann Plast Surg 2014;73(Suppl 2):S157–60.
13. Sayegh ET, Strauch RJ. Open versus endoscopic carpal tunnel release: a meta-analysis of randomized controlled trials. Clin Orthop Relat Res 2015; 473(3):1120–32.

Office-Based Percutaneous Fasciotomy for Dupuytren Contracture

James Chambers, MD, Taylor Pate, MD,
James Calandruccio, MD*

KEYWORDS

- Dupuytren contracture • Percutaneous fasciotomy • Office-based • Patient-reported outcomes

---

KEY POINTS

- Dupuytren disease is a chronic progressive disorder that affects connective tissue in various locations especially the palmar and digital fascia.
- Primary treatment goals are to completely straighten the affected ray(s) while reducing the risk of recurrence and avoiding complications.
- Minimally invasive treatment methods typically are more cost-effective, but have higher rates of recurrence compared with open procedures.
- Percutaneous fasciotomy is a safe, simple, and inexpensive treatment for mild to moderate Dupuytren contracture, with high rates of patient satisfaction and low rates of complications.

Dupuytren disease is a chronic progressive disorder that affects connective tissue in various areas and can cause functional issues when significant contractures develop in the palmar and digital fascia. The disease has an autosomal dominant inheritance pattern with variable penetrance, with family history cited as a strong predictor of the disease.[1] The disease is most commonly diagnosed in Caucasian men, with increasing prevalence in men older than 65.[1] Dupuytren disease often is tolerated for many years before the patient presents for evaluation when skin tightness and contour changes progress to form nodules, typically on the palmar aspect of the hand. These nodules produce tension in pretendinous and other cords of the palm and fingers resulting in joint flexion contractures. The contractures occur most often on the ring and small fingers with the metacarpophalangeal (MCP) and proximal interphalangeal (PIP) joints most commonly affected.[1] Treatment usually is begun for patients when the contractures are significant enough to interfere with daily activities.

Primary treatment goals are to completely straighten the affected ray(s) while reducing the risk of recurrence and avoiding complications. Treatments options are of 2 general types: minimally invasive and open surgical procedures. Minimally invasive procedures include percutaneous needle fasciotomy (PNF), cordotomy, and enzymatic fasciotomy. These options typically are more cost-effective, but have higher rates of recurrence compared with open procedures.[1,2] Open surgical procedures have higher complication rates but lower rates of recurrence and often are preferred as a second line of treatment.[1,3]

Although fasciotomy was described more than 200 years ago,[4] it was seldom used until French rheumatologists described fasciotomy with a percutaneous needle technique (PNF). The technique gained more widespread acceptance after the report by Foucher and colleagues.[5] In 2003, a series of 100 patients treated with PNF resulted in few complications, reoperation rate of 24%, and recurrence at 3-

---

Department of Orthopaedic Surgery and Biomedical Engineering, University of Tennessee-Campbell Clinic, 1211 Union Avenue, Suite 510, Memphis, TN 38104, USA
* Corresponding author.
E-mail address: jcalandruccio@campbellclinic.com

Orthop Clin N Am 51 (2020) 369–372
https://doi.org/10.1016/j.ocl.2020.02.008
0030-5898/20/© 2020 Elsevier Inc. All rights reserved.

year follow-up of 58%. More recent studies have shown that 79% of patients retain a straight joint after 2 years,[6] but recurrence of the contracture(s) remains frequent, regardless of treatment method. Pess and colleagues[7] reported a recurrence rate of 48% in 1,013 fingers followed for a median of 3 years. In their randomized controlled trial, van Rijssen and colleagues[8] found a recurrence rate of 22% with PNF compared with 5% with limited fasciectomy. Because it is a simple procedure with few complications, PNF can be done repeatedly if necessary.

The effectiveness of treatment of Dupuytren contractures can be subjectively assessed using patient-reported outcome measures (PROM). Quick Disabilities of Arm, Shoulder, and Hand (QuickDASH) is a commonly used PROM in upper extremity research including Dupuytren disease.[9] It consists of 11 questions that focus on severity of symptoms and difficulty in completing specific tasks. The QuickDASH score has 2 additional modules, work and sports/art, which focus on the patient's disability while playing a sport/musical instrument or at work. There is limited evaluation of these additional modules in patients with Dupuytren disease.

Percutaneous office-based cordotomy is an effective treatment for Dupuytren contracture; however, given that the cords are divided rather than excised, recurrence is frequent. There have been many different definitions of recurrence causing inconsistencies among studies and data, with rates ranging from 2% to 86%.[10] In 2017, Kan and colleagues[11] as part of the Dupuytren's Delphi group, addressed this problem with an expert consensus of recurrence as "an increase in extension deficit of 20° at 1 year compared to at 6 weeks post-procedure."

Identifying risk factors associated with recurrence of contracture is important because this information may change treatment plans. Degreef and De Smet,[12] in a study of more than 300 patients, showed that rates of recurrence are high for patients younger than 50 years and those with Ledderhose disease, family history, and male sex. The variable penetrance of the disease plays a confounding role in identifying specific risk factors.

Effectiveness of treatment also can be assessed from a patient's perspective using PROM. Budd and colleagues[13] showed an improvement in QuickDASH Score from 15.1 before procedure to 8.0 afterward at a mean of 110 days. The QuickDASH survey has 2 additional modules that focus on the ability to work (Work Module Score or WMS) and to play a musical instrument/sport (Sport Module Score or SMS). MacDermid and colleagues[14] studied upper extremity conditions and showed a reduction in QuickDASH score of 15 points or more to appreciate a change in function; their study, however, did not include Dupuytren disease.

The correlation between improvement of contracture and patient-reported outcomes after treatment for Dupuytren disease has been shown to be weak or nonexistent.[13,15–18] Budd and colleagues[13] showed that the change in QuickDASH score and change in extension deficit did not correlate.

Post-procedure patient satisfaction also contributes to the patient's perceived function of the digit(s). Most patients are satisfied with the outcomes of the procedure at 1 year.[6,19,20] Patient satisfaction outcomes following fasciotomy and collagenase treatment showed rates of 84% at an average of 10 months[21] and 73% at 3-year follow-up.[22]

Complication rates are low after percutaneous fasciotomy. Pess and colleagues[7] reviewed more than 1000 percutaneous releases and found skin tear to be the most common complication, occurring in only 3.4%; nerve laceration occurred in 0.1%. Skin ruptures have been reported in from 5% to 38% of patients.[20] Nerve injuries (<0.5%) and tendon injuries (<0.05%) are rare.[8,23]

PERCUTANEOUS FASCIECTOMY TECHNIQUE

- Under sterile conditions, 3.0 mL of 1% lidocaine without epinephrine is injected into the skin and subcutaneous tissues proximal to the intended site of cord division.
- A #15 scalpel blade is placed between the skin, parallel to the underlying cord (Fig. 1A).
- The finger is extended to deliver the taut cord to the blade, which is then directed perpendicular to the cord (Fig. 1B).
- The knife is gently pushed against the underlying cord with the finger held in forceful extension. The cord tissue when being divided yields a palpable gritty sensation and usually produces a predictable audible pop when the cord gives way.
- The scalpel is removed and forceful extension is used to obtain as much correction as possible (Fig. 1C).

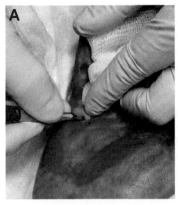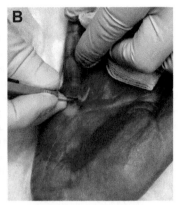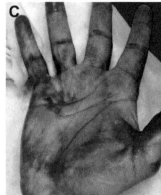

Fig. 1. (A) A #15 scalpel blade is placed between the skin, parallel to the underlying cord. (B) The finger is extended to deliver the taut cord to the blade, which is then directed perpendicular to the cord. The knife is gently pushed against the underlying cord with the finger held in forceful extension. (C) The scalpel is removed and forceful extension is used to get as much correction as possible.

- Occasionally additional sites along the cord are released, sometimes using a 25-gauge needle mounted on a syringe.

After the procedure, a soft dressing is applied and patients are instructed to begin range of motion exercises immediately. The soft dressing is removed the day after the procedure, and wound healing monitored daily for closure and home-based range-of-motion exercises are continued.

Outcomes

In 52 patients (65 digits) followed prospectively from the time of the office-based procedure to 1-year follow-up, the rate of recurrence was 33%. The average metacarpophalangeal joint correction in active extension was from 39.6° to 9.3° ($P = .001$), and passive extension correction was from 25.4° to 3.6° of hyperextension ($P = .001$). The average QuickDASH score decreased by 8, the WMS score by 12, and the SMS score by 9 compared with preoperative scores, and these decreases were statically significant. The improvement in patient-reported outcomes (WMS and SMS) did correlate at 6 weeks and 1 year with active extension improvement. Also, SMS at 1 year correlated with passive extension improvement. On average, the wound closed by 7 days and pain resolved by day 2. The average highest pain score was 2.3 on a scale of 10. None of patients who had the procedure sustained a sensory deficit. At 1 year, 82% of patients were satisfied with the outcome of their procedure, and 87% considered the procedure worth having done. A much shorter recovery time with this office-based procedure is appealing and is useful in

patients with well-defined cords, especially with MP joint contractures.

REFERENCES

1. Eaton C. Dupuytren disease. In: Wolfe SW, Hotchkiss RN, Pederson WC, et al, editors. Green's operative hand surgery. 7th edition. Philadelphia: Elsevier; 2017. p. 128–51.
2. Leafblad ND, Wagner E, Wanderman NR, et al. Outcomes and direct costs of needle aponeurotomy, collagenase injection, and fasciectomy in the treatment of Dupuytren contracture. J Hand Surg Am 2019;44:919–27.
3. Chen NC, Srinivasan RC, Shauver MJ, et al. A systematic review of outcomes of fasciotomy, aponeurotomy, and collagenase treatments for Dupuytren's contracture. Hand (N Y) 2011;6:250–5.
4. Elliot D. The early history of contracture of the palmar fascia. Part 1: the origin of the disease: the curse of the MacCrimmons: the hand of benediction: Cline's contracture. J Hand Surg Br 1988; 13:246–53.
5. Foucher G, Medina J, Navarro R. Percutaneous needle aponeurotomy: complications and results. J Hand Surg Br 2003;28:427–31.
6. Strömberg J, Ibsen-Sorensen A, Fridden J. Comparison of treatment outcome after collagenase and needle fasciotomy for dupuytren contracture: a randomized, single-blinded, clinical trial with a 1-year follow-up. J Hand Surg Am 2016;41: 873–80.
7. Pess GM, Pess RM, Pess RA. Results of needle aponeurotomy for Dupuytren contracture in over 1,000 fingers. J Hand Surg Am 2012;37:651–6.
8. van Rijssen AL, ter Linden H, Werker PM. Five-year results of a randomized clinical trial on treatment in Dupuytren's disease: percutaneous needle

fasciotomy versus limited fasciectomy. Plast Reconstr Surg 2012;129:469–77.

9. Beaton DE, Wright JG, Katz JN, et al. Development of the QuickDASH: comparison of three item-reduction approaches. J Bone Joint Surg Am 2005;87:1038–46.

10. Kan HJ, Verrijp FW, Huisstede DM, et al. The consequences of different definitions for recurrence of Dupuytren's disease. J Plast Reconstr Aesthet Surg 2013;66:95–103.

11. Kan HJ, Verrijp FW, Jouvis SER, et al. Recurrence of Dupuytren's contracture: a consensus-based definition. PLoS One 2017;12:e0164849.

12. Degreef I, De Smet L. Risk factors in Dupuytren's diathesis: is recurrence after surgery predictable? Acta Orthop Belg 2011;77:27–32.

13. Budd HR, Larson D, Chojnowski A, et al. The Quick-DASH score: a patient-reported outcome measure for Dupuytren's surgery. J Hand Ther 2011;24:15–20.

14. MacDermid JC, Richards RS, Donner A, et al. Responsiveness of the short form-36, disability of the arm, shoulder, and hand questionnaire, patient-rated wrist evaluation, and physical impairment measurements in evaluation recovery after a distal radius fracture. J Hand Surg Am 2000;25: 330–40.

15. Degreef I, Vererfve PB, De Smet L. Effect of severity of Dupuytren contracture on disability. Scand J Plast Reconstr 2009;43:41–2.

16. Engstrand C, Boren L, Liedberg GM. Evaluation of activity limitation and digital extension in Dupuytren's contracture three months after fasciectomy and hand therapy interventions. J Hand Ther 2009;22:21–6.

17. Jerosch-Herold C, Shepstone L, Chojnowski A, et al. Severity of contracture and self-reported disability in patients with Dupuytren's contracture referred for surgery. J Hand Ther 2011;24:6–10.

18. Zyluk A, Jagielski W. The effect of the severity of Dupuytren's contracture on the function of the hand before and after surgery. J Hand Surg Eur 2007;32:326–9.

19. Scherman P, Jenmalm P, Dahlin LB. One-year results of needle fasctiotomy and collagenase injection in treatment of Dupuytren's contracture: a two-centre prospective randomized clinical trial. J Hand Surg Eur 2016;41:577–82.

20. Strömberg J, Ibsen-Sorensen A, Fridden J. Percutaneous needle fasciotomy versus collagenase treatment for Dupuytren contracture: a randomized controlled trial with two-year follow-up. J Bone Joint Surg Am 2018;100:1079–86.

21. Zhou C, Hovius SE, Slijper HP, et al. Predictors of patient satisfaction with hand function after fasciectomy for Dupuytren's contracture. Plast Reconstr Surg 2016;138:649–55.

22. Bradley J, Warwick D. Patient satisfaction with collagenase. J Hand Surg Am 2016;41:689–97.

23. Krefter C, Marks M, Hensler S, et al. Complications after treating Dupuytren's disease. A systematic literature review. Hand Surg Rehabil 2017;36:322–9.

Shoulder and Elbow

Arthroscopic Latarjet for Shoulder Instability

Charles L. Getz, MD[a],*, Christopher D. Joyce, MD[b]

KEYWORDS

• Shoulder instability • Latarjet • Coracoid transfer • Arthroscopy

KEY POINTS

- Arthroscopic Latarjet offers some distinct advantages over open Latarjet, including treatment of concomitant shoulder injuries, reduced scarring and stiffness, faster recovery, and improved cosmesis.
- Indications for arthroscopic Latarjet include a failed shoulder stabilization procedure, glenoid bone loss of greater than 20%, and severe associated soft tissue injury.
- The arthroscopic Latarjet procedure is technically demanding with many steps, but after a learning curve of 20 to 25 cases, complications and speed level out.
- The current literature supports equivalent functional outcomes, recurrent instability, and complications in some series in arthroscopic versus open Latarjet procedures.

INTRODUCTION

The stability of the glenohumeral joint is provided by a number of structures. The glenohumeral joint is inherently unconstrained compared with many other joints in the human body to accommodate a large range of motion. The humeral head has a significantly larger surface area compared with the glenoid, leading to a significant portion of the humeral head being uncovered by the glenoid at any given time. This large area is one of the primary reasons that the glenohumeral joint has more motion than any other major joint in the body; however, it does also put the shoulder at risk for instability events such as dislocations or recurrent subluxations. In conjunction with the bony stability provided by the glenoid and humeral head, several soft tissue structures help to improve shoulder stability. These soft tissue structures from deep to superficial include the labrum, which is a fibrocartilagenous structure that encircles the underlying glenoid bone. The labrum functions to both deepen the socket as well as improve the congruity and negative pressure between the glenoid and humeral head to impart further stability.[1]

The glenohumeral capsule provides additional static support, particularly with the capsular thickenings that make up the superior, middle, and inferior glenohumeral ligaments and the coracohumeral ligament.[2] Further dynamic stability is provided by the rotator cuff and scapular humeral rhythm that function to balance the head in a centered position on the glenoid.[3]

Injury or failure of any of these shoulder stabilizers can lead to instability of the glenohumeral joint. During an acute anterior shoulder dislocation in a young patient, the humeral head translates anteriorly, impacting the anteroinferior glenoid. In the majority of cases, an anterior dislocation results in an anteroinferior labral tear or Bankart lesion. In other cases, the anteroinferior glenoid can fracture causing a bony Bankart lesion.[4] In the United States, most orthopedists would argue that an arthroscopic Bankart repair or a bony Bankart repair is the gold standard for surgical treatment of these injuries. A recent analysis of shoulder stabilization procedures in the United States from 2007 to 2015 showed that 87% of all instability procedures were arthroscopic Bankart repairs and only 7% were open Bankart repair.[5] This finding is

[a] Shoulder & Elbow Division, Rothman Orthopaedic Institute, 925 Chestnut Street, 5th Floor, Philadelphia, PA 19107, USA; [b] Rothman Orthopaedic Institute, 925 Chestnut Street, 5th Floor, Philadelphia, PA 19107, USA
* Corresponding author.
E-mail address: charlesgetz@hotmail.com

Orthop Clin N Am 51 (2020) 373–381
https://doi.org/10.1016/j.ocl.2020.02.002

for good reason because arthroscopic Bankart repairs have demonstrated equivalent results to open Bankart repairs in most studies while minimizing iatrogenic soft tissue damage from the open approach.[6] However, over the past decades, certain risk factors have been teased out that predispose a patient to failure in arthroscopic Bankart repair. These risk factors include younger age (<22 years), male patients, number of preoperative dislocations, participation in competitive or impact sports, fewer than 3 anchors, and glenoid or humeral bone loss.[7]

With glenoid bone loss in particular, multiple studies have found unacceptably high rates of recurrent shoulder instability after Bankart repair. Burkhart and De Beer[8] described the finding of the inverted pear–shaped glenoid that results from anteroinferior glenoid bone loss. The authors found a 67% failure rate in patients with the inverted pear glenoid compared with 4% in all other patients. In quantifying the amount of critical bone loss that will result in higher failure rates, cadaveric studies by Yamamoto and colleagues[9] and Itoi and colleagues[10] demonstrated increased risk for instability and decreased external rotation with defects larger than roughly 20%. This finding was also verified clinically in military patients by Shaha and colleagues,[11] who found a significantly higher failure rate with 20% glenoid bone loss. This study in addition to a study by Dickens and colleagues[12] suggest worse functional outcomes with bone loss as low as 13.5% in highly active patients.

It is important to identify patients with critical glenoid bone loss or other factors that predispose to Bankart repair alone. The instability severity index score is an example of a method to quantitatively identify these patients and can be used as a guideline for treatment recommendation for shoulder instability[13] (Table 1). In patients at high risk of failure of a soft tissue procedure or with prior failed instability procedures, an excellent treatment option is a coracoid process transfer or a Latarjet procedure.[14] The Latarjet procedure greatly enhances anterior glenohumeral stability by increasing the glenoid bone stock anteroinferiorly, providing a muscular sling from the lower subscapularis and conjoint tendon in abduction and external rotation, and reconstructing the anterior capsule. The open Latarjet procedure is traditionally performed through an open deltopectoral approach with a 5- to 8-cm incision and has produced excellent results overall. Two case series with more than 100 patients demonstrated recurrence instability rates as low as 2.0% to 4.9%, and overall satisfaction of 98%.[15,16] The open Latarjet procedure has also

Table 1 Description of the instability severity index score developed by Balg and colleagues	
Patient Factors	**Points**
Age, y	
<20	2
>20	0
Sport level	
Competitive	2
Recreational/none	0
Sport type	
Contact/overhead	1
Noncontact	0
Shoulder hyperlaxity	
Hyperlax	1
Normal laxity	0
Humeral bone loss	
Hill-Sachs lesion	2
No visible Hill-Sachs lesion	0
Glenoid bone loss	
Loss of glenoid contour	2
No loss of contour	0

The authors recommend against Bankart repair alone in patients with a score of >6 in favor of Latarjet.

Adapted from Balg F, Boileau P. The instability severity index score. A simple pre-operative score to select patients for arthroscopic or open shoulder stabilisation. J Bone Joint Surg Br 2007;89(11):1470-1477; with permission.

been shown to be an overall cost-effective method of treating shoulder instability.[17,18] It is also important to be aware of several other alternatives to the Latarjet procedure in cases with significant anterior glenoid bone loss. These alternatives include open or arthroscopic iliac crest autograft or distal tibial allograft glenoid reconstruction, open Bankart repair, and arthroscopic Bankart repair combined with remplissage.[19–22]

As with many procedures in orthopedic surgery, a natural evolution has developed toward more minimally invasive techniques. In the case of the Latarjet procedure, the trend was from a large open incision to a mini open incision, to now an all-arthroscopic procedure. The perceived benefits of an all-arthroscopic Latarjet procedure include visualization of the entire joint, the ability to address other pathology, less traction on the nerves of the shoulder, improved cosmesis, decreased soft tissue disruption, a lower infection rate, potentially shorter recovery times, and possibly lower complication rates. These perceived benefits are attractive to surgeons and patients alike.

INDICATIONS AND CONTRAINDICATIONS

The Latarjet procedure is indicated in several circumstances. In general, there are 2 circumstances in which a surgeon should be considering the Latarjet procedure. The first is a patient with a prior failed stabilization procedure. The second is in a patient with no prior stabilization surgery, but significant risk factors for failure of an all-soft tissue procedure such as arthroscopic Bankart repair. The primary risk factor to be included is glenoid bone loss (Fig. 1). As described previously, typically patients with at least 20% anteroinferior glenoid bone loss should be considered an indication for a Latarjet procedure. Additional patient-related risk factors should also be considered when assessing how likely a person is to fail a soft-tissue stabilization. However, it is important to note that the procedure is patient specific. The orthopedist must balance the risk of instability recurrence with other potential procedure-related complications. A summary of all indications and contraindications is included in Table 2.

SURGICAL TECHNIQUE
Preoperative Planning
Several factors play into preoperative planning. In assessing glenoid bone loss, several methods have been described. Linear glenoid bone loss or the glenoid index is best calculated by measuring the width of the diseased glenoid and dividing by the diameter of a best-fit circle on the inferior aspect of the intact contralateral glenoid.[23] Another method uses the best fit circle from the contralateral glenoid and divides the missing glenoid area by the intact contralateral area giving a better dimensional understanding of the bone loss.[24] Finally, humeral

head bone loss is assessed by the concept of the glenoid track. This system classifies lesions into on track and off track based on measuring the width of the intact glenoid and the medial extent of the Hill-Sachs lesion. Off-track lesions engage the Hill-Sachs lesion and presumably require either bone augmentation or remplissage to correct.[25] Although useful, none of these models fully consider that shoulder translation is an important component to instability.

Nonetheless, the computed tomography scan must be for 4 main factors: glenoid bone loss amount, glenoid bone loss location, humeral bone loss, and coracoid length/orientation.

1. Glenoid bone loss amount: This is calculated based on any of the methods noted elsewhere in this article. In patients with primarily glenoid bone loss, an arthroscopic Latarjet procedure alone is typically sufficient to address the pathology. However, care must be taken in extremely large defects (>30%–40% glenoid bone loss) because the coracoid transfer may not provide enough bony support to create a stable joint.
2. Glenoid bone loss location: Patients with recurrent anterior instability typically have glenoid bone loss in the anteroinferior portion of the glenoid, but this can vary anywhere from the 3 o'clock position to 6 o'clock position. It is important to note this and ensure that the coracoid transfer will fill the appropriate bone defect. Additionally, one must look for any residual nonunited bone fragments to excise to promote graft healing.
3. Humeral bone loss: Hill-Sachs lesions are extremely common in anterior shoulder instability and at times may need to be addressed. The glenoid track will still be off track, despite placement of the coracoid bone block in certain cases if the Hill-Sachs

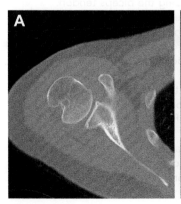 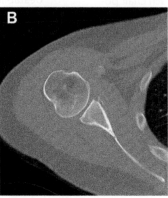

Fig. 1. Axial computed tomography scan demonstrating a (*A*) large Hill-Sachs humeral head impaction lesion with (*B*) anteroinferior glenoid bone loss in a 25-year-old man.

Table 2
Summary of the indications and contraindications to arthroscopic Latarjet

Indications	Contraindications
Failed primary instability procedure	Irreparable rotator cuff tear
Glenoid bone loss	Age >50 y
Engaging Hill-Sachs lesion	Voluntary dislocator
Irreparable anterior labrum/ capsule	Uncontrolled seizure disorder
Recurrent instability in competitive athletes	Coracoid fracture
	Coracoid insufficiency

defect is large or medial. In these cases, the surgeon should be prepared to augment stability with a remplissage or possibly even humeral head allograft.

4. Coracoid length/orientation: In considering an arthroscopic Latarjet procedure, the coracoid must be measured for its length from base to tip as well as girth. This factor is important to ensure that the graft is long enough to address the bone defect and wide enough to incorporate screws without fracture. The ideal graft is more than 25 mm long and 14 mm wide.[26] Although the coracoid length does correlate with patient height, significant variations occur based on gender and race.[27,28] Furthermore, if the coracoid base is fractured or malformed, one should not proceed with an arthroscopic Latarjet procedure.

Preparation and Patient Positioning

Our preferred position is in a low beach chair position. Either the bed backboard or an unsterile towel is placed at the medial border of the scapular to prevent scapular motion during coracoid harvest and fixation. The towel should be placed in such a manner that the scapula is positioned in a retracted position. Protraction or internal rotation of the scapula limits exposure of the anterior glenoid neck and makes proper placement of the screws more technically challenging. The patient is offered a preoperative interscalene nerve block to assist with postoperative pain. The arm is draped free to allow for repositioning during the procedure and the shoulder and chest are prepped to the midline anteriorly, the middle of the scapula posteriorly, and as inferior as the positioner devices will allow. The arm is placed in a pneumatic arm holder for the duration of the case.

Surgical Approach

The posterior portal is created in the midline of the glenohumeral joint and will be used to later guide the trajectory of the screws. The diagnostic arthroscopy is then performed, any additional pathology such as Hill-Sachs lesions, biceps tendinitis, posterior or superior labral tears, or rotator cuff tears can be visualized and addressed. A list of the typical portals used during an arthroscopic Latarjet procedure is provided in Table 3.

Surgical Procedure

- After diagnostic arthroscopy is completed, attention is first turned to the anteroinferior glenoid. In many cases, the patient will have had a failed Bankart repair or attempted glenoid rim fracture fixation. If that is the case, any suture material or screws must be removed until bare bone is exposed on the glenoid neck. This step is typically done visualizing from posterior and instrumenting through the anterior rotator interval portal.
- The glenoid neck is then prepared using an arthroscopic burr from roughly the 2 o'clock position to the 5 o'clock position. The 3 o'clock position on the glenoid is then marked with the cautery for use when positioning the graft later.
- Rotator interval tissue is then removed using an arthroscopic shaver and electrocautery. This removal must be taken all the way medially to the base of the coracoid and lateral without destabilizing the biceps tendon.
- The base of the coracoid is exposed as well as the conjoint tendon.
- An anterolateral portal is created at the upper border of the subscapularis to visualize from while instrumenting through the anterior portal.
- The superior and lateral tissues are cleared from the coracoid and conjoint tendon all of the way to the coracoclavicular ligaments superiorly and the tendon of the pectoralis major distally and lateral. A low anterior lateral portal is used for cautery and shaver to

Table 3
Summary of portals used during arthroscopic Latarjet and relative location

Portal	Location	Purpose
Posterior (A)	Posterior shoulder, in line with glenohumeral joint, 2 cm inferior to acromion	Diagnostic joint visualization
Anterior (E)	Anterior shoulder, in line with glenohumeral joint	Intra-articular instrumentation
Superior subscapularis (D)	Anterolateral portal through rotator interval, 1 cm inferior and lateral to anterolateral acromion	Anterior visualization
Midsubscapularis (J)	Midsubscapularis location between I and D portals, can be more lateral location	Straight on view of coracoid, subscapularis split
Inferior (I)	Apex of axillary fold, spinal needle directed at anteroinferior glenoid neck	Access to anteroinferior glenoid rim/neck, channeler placement
Superior coracoid (H)	Superior to coracoid, triangulation with spinal needle directed at superior coracoid	Superior coracoid instrumentation

release the pectoralis minor from the medial coracoid.

- The axillary nerve is visualized at this portion of the case. It is located medial and deep to the conjoined tendon. The musculocutaneous nerve can often be visualized after the pectoralis minor release, but is not routinely identified.
- The subscapularis tendon is then split under direct visualization by placing a switching stick through the posterior portal and directing it through the tendon. The arm is externally rotated and the switching stick is directed lateral to the conjoined tendon. Ideally, the split is about 50% from superior to inferior.
- The camera is then placed into a midanterior lateral portal to view the subscapularis en fosse. The cautery is then used through the low anterior lateral portal to split the subscapularis to its insertion on the lesser tuberosity to the musculotendinous junction.
- An accessory portal is made to allow a channeler to enter the soft tissue for future drill guide placement. This step is done by directing the posterior switching stick anterior until it is subcutaneous to identify the proper location of the channeler.
- With the camera in the midsubscapularis portal, the split is completed and the

coracoid preparation is completed by removing superior tissue to the base of the coracoid.

- Two guidewires are placed in the coracoid from an accessory portal, followed by drilling and tapping of the bone. A burr removes bone inferior, superior, and lateral on the coracoid creating a 270° osteotomy. The osteotomy is completed using an osteotome through the accessory coracoid portal.
- The coracoid graft piece is then captured using a Mitek (Warsaw, IN) guide that is threading into the previously tapped drill holes, and the undersurface of the coracoid piece is prepared with a burr. Care is taken to remove all sharp edges and have a smooth, flat back surface to allow for optimal contact with the glenoid neck.
- The graft is turned and passed between the split in the subscapularis tendon. Switching sticks from posterior can act as retractors to open the split and facilitate passing. A slight internal rotation of the arm will relax the subscapularis and make graft passage easier.
- The graft is secured onto the glenoid neck ideally between the 3 o'clock and 5 o'clock positions. The previously placed mark at the 3 o'clock position is used as a guide.

- It is then pinned and provisionally held in place with 2 wires. The 2 previously drilled screw hole act as drill guides to drill the glenoid neck. Care is taken to make the drill holes as parallel to the joint as possible. The 2 screws are then placed.
- The final graft position is checked to ensure adequate position in both the inferior–superior plane as well as the medial–lateral plane. Any overhang is removed with a burr until the graft is flush with the subchondral bone (Fig. 2).

Postoperative Rehabilitation

Postoperatively patients are placed in a sling. They are instructed to do light elbow and wrist motion exercises at home for 2 weeks. At 2 weeks, they begin passive and active assist range of motion under physical therapy guidance. At 6 weeks postoperative they, can begin active range of motion and at 12 weeks they begin strengthening. Subscapularis strength returns between 4 to 5 months from surgery and return to full activity is allowed after strength has normalized. Fig. 3 demonstrates postoperative radiographs of a well-placed coracoid transfer.

COMPLICATIONS AND MANAGEMENT

The arthroscopic Latarjet procedure is technically demanding with a relatively steep learning curve. Several studies have shown that, after about 20 to 25 cases, the learning curve begins to flatten out, which is demonstrated by decreased complications, decreased conversions to open procedure, and operative time

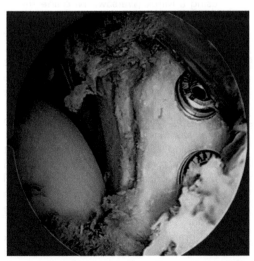

Fig. 2. Final arthroscopic view of a coracoid transfer with 2 cannulated screw fixation.

nearing that of an open Latarjet procedure.[29–31] The overall complication rate with an arthroscopic Latarjet procedure is between 6.8% and 29.0%.[30–32] Complications can be broken down into intraoperative and postoperative. Typical intraoperative complications that are documented include bone block fracture, axillary nerve palsy, and instrumentation failure requiring conversion to open. Common postoperative complications include recurrent instability, graft nonunion or resorption, symptomatic hardware, infection, stiffness, and arthritis progression.[32–35]

When comparing complication rates in arthroscopic versus open Latarjet procedures, the current literature does not provide a clear answer. Hurley and colleagues[36] in a meta-analysis found no significant difference in recurrent instability, revision rate, or overall complications when comparing open and arthroscopic Latarjet procedures, but the authors did find a significantly high rate of subjective apprehension in the arthroscopic group. Similarly, Kordasiewicz and colleagues[37] found no difference in complications, recurrent dislocation, and revision surgery rate; but, the authors did note a higher subjective apprehension in the arthroscopic group. Finally, Zhu and colleagues[38] found no difference in dislocations, complications, or apprehension between arthroscopic and open Latarjet procedures, but they did note less graft resorption in the arthroscopic patients.

OUTCOMES

Given the adequate outcomes in open Latarjet procedures, arthroscopic Latarjet procedures were scrutinized to assess for equal or improved outcomes and an acceptable complication rate in comparison. Boileau and colleagues[39] Reviewed 79 patients with arthroscopic Latarjet and Bankart repairs and found a 98% stability rate, 90% appropriate graft position, and about 9° loss of external rotation. However, the authors did find that only 73% of grafts healed radiographically with short screw length being a significant risk factor. Kany and colleagues[40] showed similar results with a 97.0% stability rate and a 91.5% appropriate graft position. In addition to these larger series of arthroscopic Latarjet procedures, several smaller case series have also demonstrated excellent results with stability up to 100% and union rates from 78% to 100%.[41–43]

In a majority of comparative studies, arthroscopic Latarjet outcomes are more or less equivalent to open Latarjet outcomes. With regard to

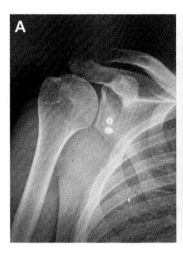 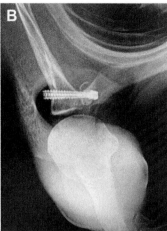

Fig. 3. Postoperative (*A*) anteroposterior and (*B*) axillary plain radiographs after an arthroscopic Latarjet procedure.

operative time, neither procedure seems to take significantly longer after the learning curve.[36] Furthermore, functional outcomes and satisfaction scores are statistically equivalent in most studies.[36,44–46] When assessing accuracy of graft position, arthroscopic Latarjet is less accurate in certain studies. Russo and colleagues[47] found that 100% of open Latarjet procedures had optimal infrequatorial graft placement, whereas only 76% of arthroscopic graft did. Neyton and colleagues[48] also found a more optimal graft position in the open Latarjet group compared with arthroscopic procedures; however, the clinical significance is unclear. In the early postoperative period (1 month), the arthroscopic Latarjet procedures do seem to have improved pain control compared with open operations.[45,46]

SUMMARY

Arthroscopic Latarjet procedures provide a less invasive option in patients with recurrent shoulder instability without any significant downsides elicited in the literature when compared with open Latarjet procedures. It is a technically demanding procedure that requires a learning curve of roughly 20 to 25 cases.

DISCLOSURE

The authors have nothing to disclose.

REFERENCES

1. Habermeyer P, Schuller U, Wiedemann E. The intra-articular pressure of the shoulder: an experimental study on the role of the glenoid labrum in stabilizing the joint. Arthroscopy 1992;8(2):166–72.

2. Turkel SJ, Panio MW, Marshall JL, et al. Stabilizing mechanisms preventing anterior dislocation of the glenohumeral joint. J Bone Joint Surg Am 1981; 63(8):1208–17.

3. Lippitt SB, Vanderhooft JE, Harris SL, et al. Glenohumeral stability from concavity-compression: A quantitative analysis. J Shoulder Elbow Surg 1993; 2(1):27–35. https://doi.org/10.1016/S1058-2746(09) 80134-1.

4. Blundell Bankart AS. Recurrent or habitual dislocation of the shoulder-joint. Br Med J 1923;2(3285): 1132–3.

5. Riff AJ, Frank RM, Sumner S, et al. Trends in shoulder stabilization techniques used in the United States based on a large private-payer database. Orthop J Sports Med 2017;5(12). 232596711774551.

6. Hobby J, Griffin D, Dunbar M, et al. Is arthroscopic surgery for stabilisation of chronic shoulder instability as effective as open surgery? A systematic review and meta-analysis of 62 studies including 3044 arthroscopic operations. J Bone Joint Surg Br 2007; 89(9):1188–96.

7. Randelli P, Ragone V, Carminati S, et al. Risk factors for recurrence after Bankart repair a systematic review. Knee Surg Sports Traumatol Arthrosc 2012; 20(11):2129–38.

8. Burkhart SS, De Beer JF. Traumatic glenohumeral bone defects and their relationship to failure of arthroscopic Bankart repairs: significance of the inverted-pear glenoid and the humeral engaging Hill-Sachs lesion. Arthroscopy 2000;16(7):677–94.

9. Yamamoto N, Itoi E, Abe H, et al. Effect of an anterior glenoid defect on anterior shoulder stability. Am J Sports Med 2009;37(5):949–54.

10. Itoi E, Lee SB, Berglund LJ, et al. The effect of a glenoid defect on anteroinferior stability of the shoulder after Bankart repair: a cadaveric study. J Bone Joint Surg Am 2000;82(1):35–46.

11. Shaha JS, Cook JB, Song DJ, et al. Redefining "critical" bone loss in shoulder instability: functional outcomes worsen with "subcritical" bone loss. Am J Sports Med 2015;43(7):1719–25.

12. Dickens JF, Owens BD, Cameron KL, et al. The effect of subcritical bone loss and exposure on recurrent instability after arthroscopic Bankart repair in intercollegiate American football. Am J Sports Med 2017;45(8):1769–75.

13. Balg F, Boileau P. The instability severity index score. J Bone Joint Surg Br 2007;89-B(11):1470–7.

14. Latarjet M. Technic of coracoid preglenoid arthroereisis in the treatment of recurrent dislocation of the shoulder. Lyon Chir 1958;54(4):604–7.

15. Hovelius L, Sandström B, Sundgren K, et al. One hundred eighteen Bristow-Latarjet repairs for recurrent anterior dislocation of the shoulder prospectively followed for fifteen years: study I - clinical results. J Shoulder Elbow Surg 2004;13(5):509–16.

16. Burkhart SS, De Beer JF, Barth JRH, et al. Results of modified Latarjet reconstruction in patients with anteroinferior instability and significant bone loss. Arthroscopy 2007;23(10):1033–41.

17. Min K, Fedorka C, Solberg MJ, et al. The cost-effectiveness of the arthroscopic Bankart versus open Latarjet in the treatment of primary shoulder instability. J Shoulder Elbow Surg 2018;27(6S):S2–9.

18. Makhni EC, Lamba N, Swart E, et al. Revision arthroscopic repair versus Latarjet procedure in patients with recurrent instability after initial repair attempt: a cost-effectiveness model. Arthroscopy 2016;32(9):1764–70.

19. Fortun CM, Wong I, Burns JP. Arthroscopic iliac crest bone grafting to the anterior glenoid. Arthrosc Tech 2016;5(4):e907–12.

20. Taverna E, Garavaglia G, Perfetti C, et al. An arthroscopic bone block procedure is effective in restoring stability, allowing return to sports in cases of glenohumeral instability with glenoid bone deficiency. Knee Surg Sports Traumatol Arthrosc 2018; 26(12):3780–7.

21. Provencher MT, Frank RM, Golijanin P, et al. Distal tibia allograft glenoid reconstruction in recurrent anterior shoulder instability: clinical and radiographic outcomes. Arthroscopy 2017; 33(5):891–7.

22. Saliken D, Lavoué V, Trojani C, et al. Combined all-arthroscopic Hill-Sachs remplissage, Latarjet, and Bankart repair in patients with bipolar glenohumeral bone loss. Arthrosc Tech 2017;6(5):e2031–7.

23. Chuang TY, Adams CR, Burkhart SS. Use of preoperative three-dimensional computed tomography to quantify glenoid bone loss in shoulder instability. Arthroscopy 2008;24(4):376–82.

24. Baudi P, Righi P, Bolognesi D, et al. How to identify and calculate glenoid bone deficit. Chir Organi Mov 2005;90(2):145–52.

25. Yamamoto N, Itoi E, Abe H, et al. Contact between the glenoid and the humeral head in abduction, external rotation, and horizontal extension: a new concept of glenoid track. J Shoulder Elbow Surg 2007;16(5):649–56.

26. Young AA, Baba M, Neyton L, et al. Coracoid graft dimensions after harvesting for the open Latarjet procedure. J Shoulder Elbow Surg 2013;22(4): 485–8.

27. Sahu D, Jagiasi J. Intraoperative and anatomic dimensions of the coracoid graft as they pertain to the Latarjet-Walch procedure. J Shoulder Elbow Surg 2019;28(4):692–7.

28. Shibata T, Izaki T, Miyake S, et al. Predictors of safety margin for coracoid transfer: a cadaveric morphometric analysis. J Orthop Surg Res 2019; 14(1):174.

29. Leuzinger J, Brzoska R, Métais P, et al. Learning curves in the arthroscopic Latarjet procedure: a multicenter analysis of the first 25 cases of 5 international surgeons. Arthroscopy 2019;35(8):2304–11.

30. Bonnevialle N, Thélu CE, Bouju Y, et al. Arthroscopic Latarjet procedure with double-button fixation: short-term complications and learning curve analysis. J Shoulder Elbow Surg 2018;27(6): e189–95.

31. Cunningham G, Benchouk S, Kherad O, et al. Comparison of arthroscopic and open Latarjet with a learning curve analysis. Knee Surg Sports Traumatol Arthrosc 2016;24(2):540–5.

32. Athwal GS, Meislin R, Getz C, et al. Short-term complications of the arthroscopic Latarjet procedure: a North American experience. Arthroscopy 2016;32(10):1965–70.

33. Haeni DL, Opsomer G, Sood A, et al. Three-dimensional volume measurement of coracoid graft osteolysis after arthroscopic Latarjet procedure. J Shoulder Elbow Surg 2017;26(3):484–9.

34. Hawi N, Reinhold A, Suero EM, et al. The anatomic basis for the arthroscopic Latarjet procedure: a cadaveric study. Am J Sports Med 2016;44(2): 497–503.

35. Lafosse T, Amsallem L, Delgrande D, et al. Arthroscopic screw removal after arthroscopic Latarjet procedure. Arthrosc Tech 2017;6(3):e559–66.

36. Hurley ET, Lim Fat D, Farrington SK, et al. Open versus arthroscopic Latarjet procedure for anterior shoulder instability: a systematic review and meta-analysis. Am J Sports Med 2019;47(5): 1248–53.

37. Kordasiewicz B, Małachowski K, Kiciński M, et al. Intraoperative graft-related complications are a risk factor for recurrence in arthroscopic Latarjet stabilisation. Knee Surg Sports Traumatol Arthrosc 2019;27(10):3230–9.

38. Zhu Y, Jiang C, Song G. Arthroscopic versus open Latarjet in the treatment of recurrent anterior

shoulder dislocation with marked glenoid bone loss: a prospective comparative study. Am J Sports Med 2017;45(7):1645–53.

39. Boileau P, Thélu C-É, Mercier N, et al. Arthroscopic Bristow-Latarjet combined with Bankart repair restores shoulder stability in patients with glenoid bone loss. Clin Orthop Relat Res 2014;472(8):2413–24.

40. Kany J, Flamand O, Grimberg J, et al. Arthroscopic Latarjet procedure: is optimal positioning of the bone block and screws possible? A prospective computed tomography scan analysis. J Shoulder Elbow Surg 2016;25(1):69–77.

41. Zhu Y-M, Jiang C, Song G, et al. Arthroscopic Latarjet procedure with anterior capsular reconstruction: clinical outcome and radiologic evaluation with a minimum 2-year follow-up. Arthroscopy 2017; 33(12):2128–35.

42. Casabianca L, Gerometta A, Massein A, et al. Graft position and fusion rate following arthroscopic Latarjet. Knee Surg Sports Traumatol Arthrosc 2016;24(2):507–12.

43. Dumont GD, Fogerty S, Rosso C, et al. The arthroscopic Latarjet procedure for anterior shoulder instability: 5-year minimum follow-up. Am J Sports Med 2014;42(11):2560–6.

44. Kordasiewicz B, Małachowski K, Kicinski M, et al. Comparative study of open and arthroscopic coracoid transfer for shoulder anterior instability (Latarjet)-clinical results at short term follow-up. Int Orthop 2017;41(5):1023–33.

45. Marion B, Klouche S, Deranlot J, et al. A prospective comparative study of arthroscopic versus mini-open Latarjet procedure with a minimum 2-year follow-up. Arthroscopy 2017;33(2):269–77.

46. Nourissat G, Neyton L, Metais P, et al. Functional outcomes after open versus arthroscopic Latarjet procedure: a prospective comparative study. Orthop Traumatol Surg Res 2016;102(8S):S277–9.

47. Russo A, Grasso A, Arrighi A, et al. Accuracy of coracoid bone graft placement: open versus arthroscopic Latarjet. Joints 2017;5(2):85–8.

48. Neyton L, Barth J, Nourissat G, et al. Arthroscopic Latarjet techniques: graft and fixation positioning assessed with 2-dimensional computed tomography is not equivalent with standard open technique. Arthroscopy 2018;34(7):2032–40.

Total Shoulder Arthroplasty Utilizing the Subscapularis-Sparing Approach

Yoav Rosenthal, MD[a], Young W. Kwon, MD, PhD[b],*

KEYWORDS

- Total shoulder arthroplasty • Subscapularis-sparing approach • Rotator interval
- Subscapularis failure

KEY POINTS

- Total shoulder arthroplasty (TSA) performed entirely through the rotator interval (or subscapularis-sparing approach) has been used in order to potentially reduce postoperative subscapularis failure.
- Patient selection is crucial to successfully perform subscapularis-sparing TSA, without jeopardizing the intact supraspinatus and subscapularis tendons.
- Although not critical, specialized instrumentation (eg, bent retractors, broach handles, and humeral component inserters) allows the subscapularis-sparing technique to be performed more efficiently and reproducibly.
- Special attention should be directed to humeral neck resection, inferior humeral neck osteophytes removal, and appropriate humeral head size selection, because these are common pitfalls of this approach.
- At any point during the procedure, if optimal visualization cannot be obtained, the procedure can be converted to the standard technique by releasing the subscapularis tendon through tenotomy, peel, or lesser-tuberosity osteotomy.

INTRODUCTION

Anatomic total shoulder arthroplasty (TSA) has been performed with high rates of patient satisfaction, decreased pain levels, and improved function to treat primary glenohumeral osteoarthritis, inflammatory arthritis, posttraumatic arthritis, and osteonecrosis of the humeral head.[1–5] Because of its efficacy, the prevalence of TSA has almost doubled in the United States in less than 10 years.[6]

Traditionally, TSA is performed through the anterior deltopectoral approach. Several methods have been described for subscapularis management in order to access the glenohumeral joint. The subscapularis tendon can be either tenotomized or peeled from the lesser tuberosity, or reflected with a lesser-tuberosity osteotomy. All 3 techniques have been described with good outcomes with none clearly demonstrating significant clinical superiority over others.[7–10] In some patients, despite advanced methods of meticulous repair, the subscapularis integrity and function may still be compromised. Subscapularis insufficiency, in turn, can lead to joint subluxation or early glenoid component loosening, resulting in patient dissatisfaction and revision surgery.[11–15]

Therefore, in 2009, Lafosse and colleagues[16] described a technique of performing the TSA procedure entirely through the rotator interval without violating the subscapularis tendon

[a] Department of Orthopaedic Surgery, Affiliated with Tel Aviv University, Rabin Medical Center, 39 Jabutinsky Road, Petah Tikva 4941492, Israel; [b] Department of Orthopaedic Surgery, New York University School of Medicine, New York University Langone Orthopedic Hospital, 301 East 17th Street, New York, NY 10003, USA
* Corresponding author.
E-mail address: young.kwon@nyulangone.org

Orthop Clin N Am 51 (2020) 383–389
https://doi.org/10.1016/j.ocl.2020.02.003
0030-5898/20/© 2020 Elsevier Inc. All rights reserved.

insertion at the lesser tuberosity. Originally, this approach used a lateral skin incision with split of the anterior and middle deltoid muscle, followed by anterior deltoid release from the acromion. According to this study,[16] the subscapularis-sparing approach yielded improved postoperative functional and pain scores as well as enhanced active range of motion and strength. Because the subscapularis tendon was never violated, this surgical approach allowed immediate postoperative active and passive range of motion, as opposed to the traditional subscapularis-violating approach, where active elevation and external rotation are restricted in the early postoperative period.

In part because of the associated technical challenges, this procedure has not yet gained wide popularity, and clinical experience with this technique is still quite limited with sparse available data in the literature. Therefore, the surgical procedure, associated technical difficulties, and early clinical data related to the subscapularis-sparing TSA are described.

OVERVIEW OF THE TECHNIQUE

The subscapularis-sparing approach can be considered for all patients with an intact rotator cuff undergoing TSA for various causes. It has been originally described by Lafosse and colleagues[16] for patients with primary osteoarthritis of the shoulder. However, the technique can also be considered for patients with posttraumatic arthritis, inflammatory arthritis, and osteonecrosis of the humeral head with associated arthritic degeneration.

The technique provides limited visualization of the glenohumeral joint. Therefore, any TSA procedure, such as revision TSA, that requires extensive manipulation of the joint would be extremely challenging and not recommended. In our experience, we also noted that the coracoid process prevents adequate exposure of the humeral head in patients with severe medial erosion of the joint due to glenoid bone loss. Similarly, in obese patients or those with large anterior deltoid muscle, the glenoid exposure through the rotator interval can be compromised. Therefore, severe glenoid bone loss, obesity, and large anterior deltoid muscle mass are relative contraindications and not recommended for those surgeons unfamiliar with the technique (Box 1). It should also be noted that, at any point during the procedure, the subscapularis can be released and the procedure can be converted to the standard technique. Therefore, surgeons can gain experience with this

---

Box 1
Surgical indications and contraindications

Indications

Considered for all total shoulder arthroplasty candidates with:

- Glenohumeral arthritis
- Posttraumatic arthritis
- Inflammatory arthritis
- Osteonecrosis of the humeral head

Relative contraindications:

- Severe medial erosion of the joint due to glenoid bone loss
- Obese patients
- Large anterior deltoid mass

---

technique even when the entire TSA procedure cannot be performed as initially planned.

Because of the limited surgical exposure, the subscapularis-sparing TSA is technically more demanding and likely requires a steep "learning curve." However, with experience, the technique can be performed efficiently. Thus, according to Ding and colleagues,[17] in comparison to the standard TSA technique using subscapularis tenotomy, the subscapularis-sparing approach did not require significantly longer operative time (124 minutes vs 117 minutes, $P = .17$).

SURGICAL TECHNIQUE
Preparation/Patient Positioning

A standard set of radiographs with perpendicular views of the joint is required to clearly visualize and assess the joint for any deformities, including bone loss (Fig. 1). In addition, most

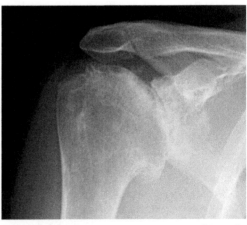

Fig. 1. Preoperative anteroposterior view plain radiograph of the shoulder.

surgeons also routinely obtain computed tomographic scans with 3-dimentional reconstruction images to quantify the degree of glenoid bone loss and version.

The patient is positioned in a manner that is typical for all TSA. Thus, most are placed in a "beach chair" position with the torso in about 30° to 45° of flexion. The head and neck should be secured, and the trunk should be stabilized in order to accurately estimate the glenoid version during the procedure. In addition, the arm must be allowed to fully extend in order to provide complete humeral head exposure.

Surgical Approach

Unlike the original description by Lafosse and colleagues,[16] the subscapularis-sparing approach has been modified and utilizes an anterior deltopectoral approach. Hence, the modified approach does not violate the deltoid and improves access to the inferior neck osteophytes.[18] The surgical incision is established anteriorly, about 1 to 1.5 cm lateral to tip of the coracoid, extending distally parallel to the standard deltopectoral skin incision. After establishing skin flaps, the deltopectoral interval is identified and developed to expose the joint.

The inferior 5 to 7 mm of the subscapularis insertion at the humeral neck, which is mostly muscular, is split parallel to its fibers to visualize the inferior capsule. Despite partially splitting and elevating the inferior portion of the subscapularis, the superior portion the tendon remains intact, maintaining its mechanical strength.[19] Through this "window" in the inferior subscapularis, the inferior capsule is excised and the inferior humeral neck osteophytes are removed (Fig. 2). Extra caution must be taken during this portion of the procedure to avoid injuring the nearby neurovascular structures.

The proximal portion of the long head of the biceps tendon must be mobilized such that the bicipital groove can clearly be identified. Although it is not necessary, most surgeons choose to perform a soft tissue biceps tendon tenodesis against the pectoralis major tendon and resect the proximal portion of the long head of biceps tendon. Subsequently, the shoulder is extended, and the bicipital groove is used to identify the rotator interval. The rotator interval is split parallel to the subscapularis, and the exposure is extended by excising all the soft tissue within the rotator interval (Fig. 3).

By inserting appropriate retractors, the humeral head can then be visualized for resection (Fig. 4A, B). The anterior and posterior borders of the native humeral head can be used as a

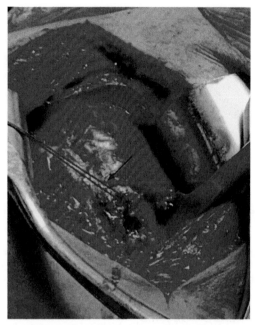

Fig. 2. The inferior 5 to 7 mm of the subscapularis insertion is split, parallel to its fibers (*arrow*) to expose and excise the inferior capsule, held by a suture (*asterisk*). This allows adequate visualization and proper removal of the inferior humeral neck osteophytes.

reference to determine the angle of the humeral cut. Alternatively, an extramedullary cutting guide can also be attached to the bicipital groove. It should be noted, however, that for

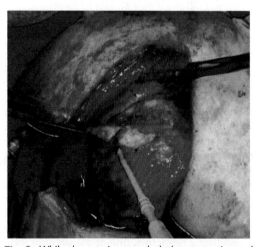

Fig. 3. While the arm is extended, the rotator interval is split parallel to the superior border of the subscapularis tendon (*asterisk*), and the soft tissue within the interval is excised. Caution is taken to avoid damaging the anterior margin of the supraspinatus tendon (*arrow*).

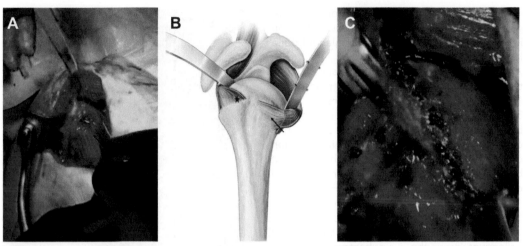

Fig. 4. (A, B) The humeral head is visualized by inserting appropriate retractors about the supraspinatus (*asterisk*) and the subscapularis (*arrow*) tendons. (C) Following determination of the humeral neck cut angle, the humeral head is resected using a narrow blade microsagittal saw. ([B] *Courtesy of* Exactech, Inc., Gainesville, FL.)

the cutting guide in the bicipital groove to be effective, any residual osteophytes about the groove must be resected entirely. The humeral head cut is initiated with a narrow blade microsagittal saw because a standard sized blade can potentially damage the supraspinatus or the subscapularis tendon insertions (Fig. 4C). After establishing the initial cut in the bone, straight osteotomes are then used to complete the cut and remove the humeral head. Any residual osteophytes about the humeral head are then removed through the rotator interval.

Bone Preparation and Insertion of Prostheses

At this stage in the procedure, attention can be directed either to the glenoid or to the humeral canal at the surgeon's typical preference. In order to obtain optimal exposure of the glenoid, the anterior lateral soft tissues, including the anterior deltoid muscle, must be retracted posteriorly. Therefore, in obese patients or those with large anterior deltoid muscle mass (eg, young men), the glenoid exposure may be compromised. For most patients, the humerus should be retracted slightly inferiorly and posteriorly. Because of the confined and limited space provided by the rotator interval, additional retractors do not necessarily provide improved exposure. In fact, for optimal exposure, we found that 2 retractors, one at the anterior inferior glenoid rim and another at the posterior inferior quadrant, are generally sufficient and preferred. After adequate soft tissue releases, the glenoid is prepared (Fig. 5), and the prosthesis is inserted.

After inserting the glenoid prosthesis, the arm is placed in adduction and extension to expose the proximal humerus through the rotator interval. The humeral canal is prepared (Fig. 6), and the humeral head eccentricity and size are confirmed. Because of the limited exposure through the rotator interval, this portion of the procedure can be challenging. In patients with medial erosion of the joint due to glenoid bone loss, the lateral edge of the coracoid process will interfere with the surgical field. If needed, intraoperative fluoroscopy can be helpful to confirm the size and coverage with the humeral head trial component.

Once the final humeral head size is determined, trial components are removed, and the

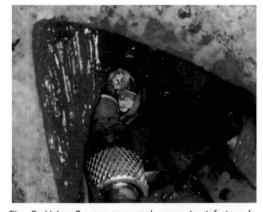

Fig. 5. Using 2 retractors at the anterior-inferior glenoid rim and at the posterior-inferior quadrant, the glenoid surface is exposed and prepared with drilling and sequential reaming.

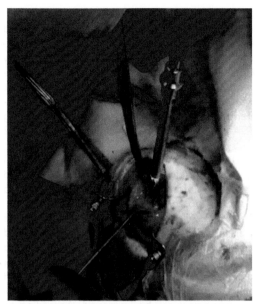

Fig. 6. Maintaining arm adduction and extension, the humeral canal is prepared with sequential reaming and broaching.

final implants are assembled on the back table. Using a low-profile humeral insertion device, the humeral prosthesis is inserted into the humeral canal and rotated into the appropriate position under the supraspinatus tendon (Fig. 7). After allowing the humeral head to sink underneath the supraspinatus, the component is finally impacted and seated. The rotator interval is then closed with side-to-side repair of the upper subscapularis to the anterior supraspinatus using heavy nonabsorbable sutures (Fig. 8). This repair should be avoided within 1.5 cm of the coracoid base because the coracohumeral ligament may

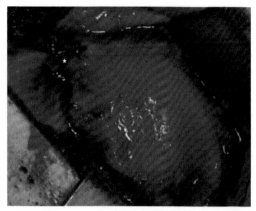

Fig. 8. Side-to-side repair of the upper subscapularis tendon to the anterior supraspinatus tendon is performed to close the rotator interval (*asterisk*).

be excessively tightened and limit postoperative external rotation. Before transferring the patient to recovery, shoulder plain radiographs are taken to ensure joint congruency and assess component positioning (Fig. 9).

Postoperative Rehabilitation
Although a sling is provided for comfort, patients are directed to wear the sling at their discretion. Passive and active motion exercises are initiated immediately after the surgery without limitations. Resistive training and shoulder girdle musculature strengthening exercises are generally initiated 6 to 8 weeks after surgery.

CLINICAL OUTCOME

TSA, performed through a subscapularis-sparing approach, provides significantly decreased pain

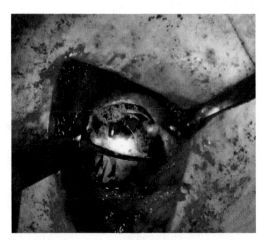

Fig. 7. The humeral prosthesis is inserted into the canal under the supraspinatus tendon, rotated to the appropriate position and finally impacted and seated.

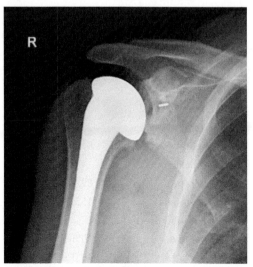

Fig. 9. Postoperative anteroposterior view plain radiograph of the replaced shoulder.

levels, improved function, and improved active range of motion in most patients. For example, Lafosse and colleagues[16] examined patients treated with the subscapularis-sparing approach at an average of 28.6 months postoperatively and reported improved outcome and pain. As such, the constant score improved by a mean of 43.3 (from 25.1 to 68.5); visual analogue scale (VAS) score decreased by a mean of 5.7 (from 8.1 to 2.4); simple shoulder test score improved by 70.7 (from 16.1 to 86.8), and active forward flexion improved by 77° (from 71.2° to 148.2°).

Similarly, Kwon and Zuckerman[18] analyzed 32 patients treated with this technique at a minimum of 2-year follow-up and reported improved VAS from 6.6 ± 2.1 to 1.6 ± 2.2 and American Shoulder and Elbow Surgeons (ASES) scores from 29.3 ± 12.5 to 81.7 ± 23.3. Active forward flexion and external rotation also improved in these patients from 89.5° ± 28.3° and 15.8° ± 12.6° to 155.8 ± 23.3° and 46.0° ± 11.5°, respectively. Kwon and Zuckerman also compared this group of patients against 38 patients who were treated with the standard TSA technique using the subscapularis tenotomy. At this short-term follow-up, all outcome measurements, including VAS, ASES score, active elevation, and external rotation, were similar in both groups with no statistically significant differences. Complication and reoperation rates were also similar in the 2 groups (Table 1).

In addition to promising clinical results, Lafosse and colleagues[16] also noted in their original report that all patients treated with the subscapularis-sparing technique maintained subscapularis integrity as evidenced by negative belly press test. In a separate study by Routman and Savoie,[20] MRI and ultrasonography demonstrated an intact subscapularis, without evidence of muscular atrophy, in all patients who underwent a subscapularis-sparing TSA at a short- to medium-term follow-up of 2 to 5 years.

Using the original surgical technique with the lateral skin incision and anterior deltoid release, Lafosse and colleagues[16] found notable postoperative radiographic errors. They noted that the humeral neck osteotomies were nonanatomic in 35% (6/17); humeral head implants were undersized in 29% (5/17), and 47% (8/17) retained inferior humeral neck osteophytes. By modifying the technique and using the deltopectoral approach, these radiographic errors can be improved. According to Ding and colleagues,[17] in comparison to standard subscapularis tenotomy technique, patients treated with subscapularis-sparing technique TSA demonstrated similar recreation of the shoulder anatomy. However, patients treated with the subscapularis-sparing TSA technique also demonstrated a greater tendency to maintain larger (>4 mm) humeral neck osteophytes. With the available sample size, it was unclear whether these radiographic errors were associated with inferior clinical outcomes.

Table 1
Preoperative and postoperative scores and range of motion in the subscapularis-sparing versus the standard groups of patients

| Outcome Parameter | Mean ± Standard Deviation | | P Value |
	Subscapularis-Sparing Group	Standard Group	
VAS score			
Preoperative	6.6 ± 2.1	6.3 ± 2.4	.628
Postoperative	1.6 ± 2.2	1.0 ± 1.7	.188
ASES score			
Preoperative	29.3 ± 12.5	32.8 ± 16.1	.328
Postoperative	81.7 ± 23.3	87.1 ± 14.5	.290
Forward flexion			
Preoperative	89.5°±28.3°	88.0°±29.9°	.829
Postoperative	155.8°±23.3°	154.6°±21.7°	.848
External rotation			
Preoperative	15.8°±12.6°	14.7°±16.9°	.771
Postoperative	46.0°±11.5°	52.1°±20.8°	.219

Data from Kwon YW, Zuckerman JD. Subscapularis-Sparing Total Shoulder Arthroplasty: A Prospective, Double-Blinded, Randomized Clinical Trial. Orthopedics 2019;42(1):e61-e67.

SUMMARY

Subscapularis integrity and function are crucial to achieve and retain successful clinical outcome following TSA. Several methods to manage the subscapularis tendon during TSA have been described. However, none appear to be clinically superior in minimizing postoperative subscapularis dysfunction. Performing TSA entirely through the rotator interval has the potential benefit of accelerated rehabilitation and avoids subscapularis failure. Large-number series and long-term follow-up are still required to determine the importance of this approach.

DISCLOSURE

The authors have nothing to disclose.

REFERENCES

1. Norris TR, Iannotti JP. Functional outcome after shoulder arthroplasty for primary osteoarthritis: a multicenter study. J Shoulder Elbow Surg 2002;11: 130–5.
2. Neyton L, Kirsch JM, Collotte P, et al. Mid- to long-term follow-up of shoulder arthroplasty for primary glenohumeral osteoarthritis in patients aged 60 or under. J Shoulder Elbow Surg 2019;28:1666–73.
3. Patel RB, Muh S, Okoroha KR, et al. Results of total shoulder arthroplasty in patients aged 55 years or younger versus those older than 55 years: an analysis of 1135 patients with over 2 years of follow-up. J Shoulder Elbow Surg 2019;28:861–8.
4. Favard L, Katz D, Colmar M, et al. Total shoulder arthroplasty–arthroplasty for glenohumeral arthropathies: results and complications after a minimum follow-up of 8 years according to the type of arthroplasty and etiology. Orthop Traumatol Surg Res 2012;98:S41–7.
5. Deshmukh AV, Koris M, Zurakowski D, et al. Total shoulder arthroplasty: long-term survivorship, functional outcome, and quality of life. J Shoulder Elbow Surg 2005;14:471–9.
6. Dillon MT, Chan PH, Inacio MCS, et al. Yearly trends in elective shoulder arthroplasty, 2005-2013. Arthritis Care Res (Hoboken) 2017;69:1574–81.
7. Lapner PL, Sabri E, Rakhra K, et al. Comparison of lesser tuberosity osteotomy to subscapularis peel in shoulder arthroplasty: a randomized controlled trial. J Bone Joint Surg Am 2012;94:2239–46.
8. Shields E, Ho A, Wiater JM. Management of the subscapularis tendon during total shoulder arthroplasty. J Shoulder Elbow Surg 2017;26:723–31.
9. Choate WS, Kwapisz A, Momaya AM, et al. Outcomes for subscapularis management techniques in shoulder arthroplasty: a systematic review. J Shoulder Elbow Surg 2018;27:363–70.
10. Aibinder WR, Bicknell RT, Bartsch S, et al. Subscapularis management in stemless total shoulder arthroplasty: tenotomy versus peel versus lesser tuberosity osteotomy. J Shoulder Elbow Surg 2019; 28:1942–7.
11. Moeckel BH, Altchek DW, Warren RF, et al. Instability of the shoulder after arthroplasty. J Bone Joint Surg Am 1993;75:492–7.
12. Miller SL, Hazrati Y, Klepps S, et al. Loss of subscapularis function after total shoulder replacement: a seldom recognized problem. J Shoulder Elbow Surg 2003;12:29–34.
13. Miller BS, Joseph TA, Noonan TJ, et al. Rupture of the subscapularis tendon after shoulder arthroplasty: diagnosis, treatment, and outcome. J Shoulder Elbow Surg 2005;14:492–6.
14. Caplan JL, Whitfield B, Neviaser RJ. Subscapularis function after primary tendon to tendon repair in patients after replacement arthroplasty of the shoulder. J Shoulder Elbow Surg 2009;18:193–6 [discussion: 7–8].
15. Gerber C, Yian EH, Pfirrmann CA, et al. Subscapularis muscle function and structure after total shoulder replacement with lesser tuberosity osteotomy and repair. J Bone Joint Surg Am 2005;87:1739–45.
16. Lafosse L, Schnaser E, Haag M, et al. Primary total shoulder arthroplasty performed entirely thru the rotator interval: technique and minimum two-year outcomes. J Shoulder Elbow Surg 2009;18:864–73.
17. Ding DY, Mahure SA, Akuoko JA, et al. Total shoulder arthroplasty using a subscapularis-sparing approach: a radiographic analysis. J Shoulder Elbow Surg 2015;24:831–7.
18. Kwon YW, Zuckerman JD. Subscapularis-sparing total shoulder arthroplasty: a prospective, double-blinded, randomized clinical trial. Orthopedics 2019;42:e61–7.
19. Simovitch RW, Nayak A, Scalise J, et al. Biomechanical characteristics of subscapularis-sparing approach for anatomic total shoulder arthroplasty. J Shoulder Elbow Surg 2018;27:133–40.
20. Routman HD, Savoie FHB. Subscapularis-sparing approaches to total shoulder arthroplasty: ready for prime time? Clin Sports Med 2018;37:559–68.

Foot and Ankle

Minimally Invasive Achilles Repair Techniques

Thomas Clanton, MD[a], Ingrid K. Stake, MD[b],*, Katherine Bartush, MD[c], Marissa D. Jamieson, MD[c]

KEYWORDS

- Achilles rupture • Achilles repair • Minimally invasive • Mini-open
- Percutaneous Achilles Repair System (PARS) • Achilles Midsubstance SpeedBridge

---

KEY POINTS

- Minimally invasive surgical techniques for acute Achilles tendon ruptures have demonstrated low complication rates and comparable functional outcomes to open techniques.
- The newer minimally invasive technique, the Achilles Midsubstance SpeedBridge repair, is a knotless technique using the PARS device for suturing the tendon proximally and bone anchors for fixing the sutures distally into the calcaneus.
- Preliminary results with Achilles Midsubstance SpeedBridge repair have been promising with satisfactory outcome and early return to sports.

INTRODUCTION

The incidence of Achilles tendon rupture has increased over the last decades.[1,2] It is now the most common tendon rupture of the lower extremity with a reported incidence of 21.5 per 100,000 person-years in 2011.[1,3] The highest incidence is reported in men in their fourth and fifth decades of life, but the mean age is increasing.[1,2,4]

Because the Achilles tendon is the most important plantar flexor of the foot, rupture can have a significant impact on function. The goal of treatment is to restore tendon integrity and length so that the patient can return to full activity with preinjury strength.[5] Although the optimal treatment is debated, both conservative treatment with early functional rehabilitation and surgical management have achieved good outcomes.[6] Recent comparative studies have reported limited differences between operative and nonoperative management with comparable rerupture rates and only a small difference in plantar flexion strength in favor of operative treatment.[6–8]

Although successful results after nonoperative treatment have been reported, there may still be a risk for tendon elongation, muscle weakness, prolonged rehabilitation, and delayed return to activities.[6–11] It has been suggested that studies comparing nonoperative and operative treatment may not be adequately powered to detect a clinically significant difference in outcome.[5,11] The assumed difference may be a concern, especially in athletes with high demands on ankle function. In this patient population, surgical treatment is still the recommended treatment of choice.

Open surgical treatment has been the standard for treating acute Achilles tendon ruptures using a Krackow suture technique.[12] This Krackow suture technique directly brings the ruptured tendon ends together, allowing for healing with high-quality tissue, thereby reducing the risk of rerupture.[9] The disadvantage of this technique is the high risk of complications, including infection, wound-healing problems, sural nerve injuries, and scar complaints.[9,13,14] Excluding

---

[a] Foot and Ankle Sports Medicine, The Steadman Clinic and Steadman Philippon Research Institute, 181 West Meadow Drive, Suite 400, Vail, CO 81657, USA; [b] Department of Orthopaedic Surgery, Ostfold Hospital Trust, Norway and Steadman Philippon Research Institute, 181 West Meadow Drive, Suite 400, Vail, CO 81657, USA; [c] Steadman Philippon Research Institute, 181 West Meadow Drive, Suite 400, Vail, CO 81657, USA
* Corresponding author.
E-mail address: istake@sprivail.org

reruptures, a total complication risk of 34% has been reported, compared with 3% after nonoperative treatment.[13]

To reduce the risk of complications associated with open surgery, less-invasive surgical techniques have been introduced. The first percutaneous technique was reported by Ma and Griffith[15] in 1977. This technique included medial and lateral stab incisions and suture of the ruptured tendon with a Bunnell suture proximally and a box suture distally. Even though they reported promising results, subsequent studies reported mixed rates of sural nerve injuries with rates up to 16.7%.[16] In a metaanalysis involving 800 patients, percutaneous techniques demonstrated a reduction in reruptures and overall complication rate compared with open surgical techniques.[13]

To better ensure approximation of the tendon ends and reduce the risk of complications, an approach combining the properties of the open and percutaneous techniques is preferred.[17] Several minimally invasive techniques have been described. Elton and Bluman[18] reported a technique using curved ring forceps to grasp the Achilles tendon and pass sutures through. In a case series of 100 consecutive cases that underwent a small proximal medial incision and suture with the Dresden technique, there was 98% patient satisfaction, no cases of sural nerve injury or wound complications, and only 2 patients with reruptures.[19] A technique by Kakiuchi[17] used a suture guide made of Kirschner wires for assistance in suturing the tendon ends that also made it possible to pull the sutures inside the paratenon and avoid sural nerve entrapment. In 12 patients, the results demonstrated fewer symptoms, better single-limb hopping, and higher return to sports compared with open surgery at mean 5.1 years postoperatively.

The technique by Kakiuchi and colleagues[17] was the precursor for the Achillon device (Integra Life Science Corporation, Plainsboro, NJ, USA), which was first reported on in 2002.[20] This device was designed to facilitate a better and more standardized technique for suturing Achilles tendon ruptures. Prospective studies have shown that repair with the Achillon device has equivalent outcomes to open repairs with lower complication rates, including fewer wound problems.[21,22] A metaanalysis reported fewer wound complications with the Achillon device and no differences in rerupture rate, sural nerve injury, return to sports, or American Orthopaedic Foot and Ankle Society (AOFAS) score compared with open repair.[21] A biomechanical

suture study compared the Achillon device, a 4-strand Krackow, and a 4-strand Krackow with augmented suture and reported earlier failure with the Achillon device caused by suture pullout through the tendon.[23]

Since 2010, the Percutaneous Achilles Repair System (PARS, Arthrex, Inc, Naples, FL) has been available. This device is similar to the Achillon device, but includes nonlocking and locking sutures to better grasp the tendon ends and potentially improve the strength of the repair, allowing for earlier mobilization.[24] The device allows for 3 sutures to be passed through each end of the rupture, and the corresponding sutures are tied.

A knotless technique has recently been developed, whereby the PARS device is used proximally to suture the tendon, and bone anchors are used distally to fix the sutures to the calcaneal bone.[25] This technique, the Achilles Midsubstance SpeedBridge repair (Arthrex, Inc, Naples, FL, USA), avoids the risk of failure at the knots and suture cutout from the distal part of the tendon, which has been reported with the PARS technique.[24,26] In addition, the lack of knots allows for better respect of the soft tissue envelope at the rupture site and the musculotendinous length to be set intraoperatively.[25] A biomechanical study resulted in a modification of the initial technique, and SutureTape (Arthrex, Inc) is now the preferred suture.[26] The Achilles Midsubstance SpeedBridge repair has shown promising results and is the authors' preferred surgical method for Achilles tendon ruptures.

INDICATIONS/CONTRAINDICATIONS

The indication for surgical treatment with the Achilles Midsubstance SpeedBridge system is acute Achilles tendon rupture in athletes or active patients.[27] Conservative treatment may be preferred in older patients, especially if comorbidities resulting in higher risk of wound complications are present. Contraindications include chronic ruptures (more than 6 weeks old), previous surgery of the Achilles tendon, and open ruptures.[28]

SURGICAL TECHNIQUE/PROCEDURE
Preparation and Patient Positioning
The patient is placed under anesthesia, and a thigh tourniquet is applied. Next, the patient is placed in the prone position, and all bony prominences are well padded. It is important to assess the resting tension, or carrying angle, of the nonoperative Achilles. The feet should be off

of the bed with a small bolster under the affected side. The bolster facilitates suture passage by removing the contralateral limb from the area needed to pass suture. Be sure the operative extremity is not rotated; if so, a nonsterile bump can be placed under the lateral thigh. Some surgeons prefer to include the nonoperative lower extremity in the sterile field, but this is unnecessary if the surgeon has a clear memory of the natural flexion angle of the uninjured ankle.

Surgical Approach

Exsanguinate the limb and inflate the tourniquet. Begin by palpating the defect in the Achilles. Make a 3-cm transverse incision approximately 1 cm proximal to the defect (Fig. 1). A transverse incision disrupts the paratenon less than a longitudinal incision. Be cautious of the sural nerve laterally.

A longitudinal incision allows for an extensile approach and may be needed in cases of tendinosis, calcifications, or chronic tendon tears. Alternatively, one can extend the incision in an L- or Z-shaped fashion. Be aware of the sural nerve in the lateral aspect of the incision. Use blunt dissection to define and protect the nerve with a vessel loop or continuous blunt retraction.

Next, use sharp dissection to expose the paratenon. Incise the paratenon in a transverse fashion parallel to the skin incision and preserve this for repair at the conclusion of the procedure. Place 2 small Kocher clamps, one medially and one laterally, on the distal end of the proximal Achilles stump. If the injury is not acute, mobilization of the tendon will be required. Therefore, release adhesions from the dorsal, medial, and lateral portion of tendon with a Freer elevator or ribbon malleable retractor (Fig. 2). Avoid dissection anterior to the tendon to protect its blood supply.

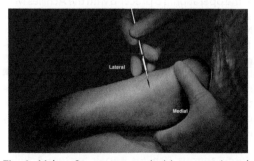

Fig. 1. Make a 3-cm transverse incision approximately 1 cm proximal to the defect. (*From* Liechti DJ, Moatshe G, Backus JD, et al. A Percutaneous Knotless Technique for Acute Achilles Tendon Ruptures. Arthrosc Tech 2018;7(2):e172; with permission.)

Instrumentation

On the back table, dial the jig's inner arms to their narrowest position. Then, widen them with the center turn wheel inside the paratenon so they can capture the tendon. Being inside the paratenon helps protect the sural nerve. While retracting the tendon distally with the Kocher clamps, insert the jig as far proximally as it will go (Fig. 3). The jig should slide without resistance, and the suture retrieval hooks next to the proximal stump will be stopped by the gastrocnemius-soleus-complex muscle belly. Palpate proximally and assess the handle. It should be parallel to the ground to ensure that the arms are in line with the tendon. The most common mistake is to have the handle pointing up, which leaves the arms of the jig deep to the tendon.

Suture Passage

Begin by identifying the numbered holes in the jig. The corresponding wires are 1.6 mm in size and have nitinol loops on the end. They will first be used without the corresponding suture before passing. Provisionally, fix the jig proximally by placing the first needle in the number 1 hole without its suture and leaving it in place (Fig. 4).

Place the second needle through hole number 2 and shuttle a blue and white–striped SutureTape across the tendon. Place needles number 3 and number 4. They are oriented in oblique directions and form the locking construct; number 3 is oriented from superior to inferior, whereas number 4 is oriented from inferior to superior. Shuttle a green and white–striped SutureTape with a loop on each end so that the loops are on opposite sides of the lower leg (Fig. 5).

A black and white–striped SutureTape is passed through the number 5 hole. Return to the first wire and shuttle a white SutureTape through the first hole. Holes number 6 and number 7 are optional for a second locking suture.

Turn the center wheel to narrow the arms. Slide the jig distally out of the wound while managing the suture on each side of the tendon (Fig. 6). Suture management is a key to making the procedure proceed smoothly. Use a hemostat to gently deliver each loop of sutures from the wound. Test them for security by gently pulling distally on them. If the tendon is not secure, remove the sutures and begin again at the first hole.

Suture Locking

To emphasize, suture management is the key to making suture locking as smooth as possible. Arrange the sutures outside of the wound bed

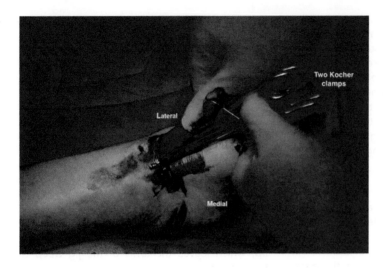

Fig. 2. Place 2 small Kocher clamps, one medially and one laterally, on the distal end of the proximal Achilles stump. Release adhesions from the dorsal, medial, and lateral portion of tendon with a ribbon malleable retractor. (*Adapted from* Liechti DJ, Moatshe G, Backus JD, et al. A Percutaneous Knotless Technique for Acute Achilles Tendon Ruptures. Arthrosc Tech 2018;7(2):e172; with permission.)

in the following order (Fig. 7): white SutureTape, blue and white–striped SutureTape, 1 green and white–striped suture with loop lateral, 1 green and white–striped suture with loop medial, and most distally, black and white–striped Suture-Tape. Pass the blue and white–striped Suture-Tape into the loop on each side by first taking the SutureTape underneath, wrap it around the green and white sutures twice, and place it through the loop. This suturing method will be done with the blue and white suture limb on the lateral side, and the blue and white suture limb on the medial side. When the suture wraps are complete, pull on the nonlooped side of the green and white sutures on each side of the leg and remove the green and white sutures from the field. This method locks the blue and white SutureTape within the tendon, and the construct now consists of 2 nonlocking SutureTapes and 1 locking SutureTape on each side of the tendon (Figs. 8–11). Precondition the sutures by placing maximum axial tension on each suture individually for 10 cycles. Cycling of the proximal stump sutures will prevent suture creep postoperatively and ensure that each suture captures the proximal tendon stump. If a suture pulls out of the proximal tendon, it was not secure enough to be functional, and an attempt can be made to replace proximal sutures by replacing the PARS device. As an alternative, the PARS can be abandoned, and the procedure can be converted to a traditional open procedure by turning the transverse incision into a Z-shaped incision.

The steps of the PARS and Achilles Midsubstance SpeedBridge are the same up to this point in the operation. To proceed with the Achilles Midsubstance SpeedBridge, proceed to step "Achilles Midsubstance SpeedBridge" in later discussion. To continue with the PARS technique, place a hemostat onto the 3 medial and another onto the 3 lateral sutures. Then, repeat the abovementioned steps for the distal aspect of the tendon. Be sure to insert the jig as distal as possible. Again, precondition these sutures by individually pulling axial traction on them.

Percutaneous Achilles Repair System Achilles Tensioning and Suture Tying

Remove any slack from the sutures before tying. The authors have found it is virtually impossible to overtension this repair; therefore, place the

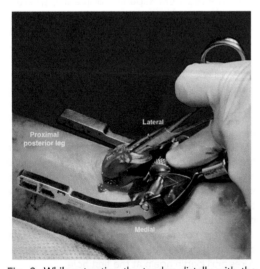

Fig. 3. While retracting the tendon distally with the Kocher clamps, insert the jig as far proximally as it will go. (*Adapted from* Liechti DJ, Moatshe G, Backus JD, et al. A Percutaneous Knotless Technique for Acute Achilles Tendon Ruptures. Arthrosc Tech 2018;7(2):e172; with permission.)

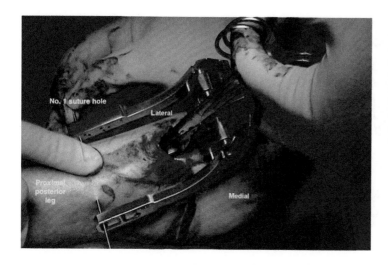

Fig. 4. Provisionally, fix the jig proximally by placing the first needle in the number 1 hole without its suture and leaving it in place. (*Adapted from* Liechti DJ, Moatshe G, Backus JD, et al. A Percutaneous Knotless Technique for Acute Achilles Tendon Ruptures. Arthrosc Tech 2018;7(2):e172; with permission.)

operative ankle in plantar flexion during knot tying approximately 15° more plantarflexed than the uninvolved ankle. In order to preserve the resting tension, either have an assistant to pull traction on the poststrand or place a hemostat on the knot before it is locked. The natural elongation that occurs during the first months postoperatively will result in the resting tension of the ankle to end up in a similar position as the uninvolved ankle.

After the wound has been irrigated, be sure that the knots are buried and will not irritate the subcutaneous tissue. Close the paratenon

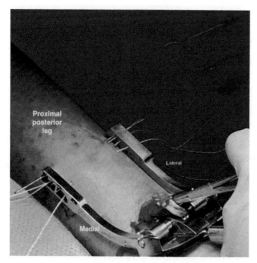

Fig. 5. Shuttle a green and white–striped SutureTape with loop on each end so that the loops are on opposite sides of the lower leg. (This image provided courtesy of Arthrex®, Naples, Florida 2020.)

with absorbable suture. The authors prefer 3.0 Monocryl sutures in the subcutaneous tissue and horizontal 4.0 nylon sutures for the skin.

Achilles Midsubstance SpeedBridge

Incise the posterior aspect of the heel at the level of the Achilles insertion to the calcaneus with 4- to 5-mm longitudinal incisions on each side of the calcaneus. These incisions should be distal to the convex surface of the posterior calcaneus. Using a soft tissue sleeve, make a 3.5-mm drill hole in each of these incisions, followed by the 4.75-mm tap. This hole should aim toward the midline at an angle approximately 45° from the tendon and be at least 19 mm in depth. Place a guide pin in these 2 bone holes to preserve their location during the next steps.

A Banana SutureLasso (Arthrex, Inc) is then passed through each incision in a retrograde direction (Fig. 12); this will emerge through the previous transverse incision. Use the Banana SutureLasso to pass the medial and lateral 3 sutures through the lower stump and out of the ipsilateral calcaneal incisions.

Load the respective sutures onto a 4.75-mm BioComposite SwiveLock anchor and place them into the calcaneal holes (Fig. 13). While turning the paddle so, be sure to pull axial traction and exceed the equinus of the nonoperative ankle by approximately 15°. If both limbs are in the sterile field with a bolster, the bolsters should be the same size. Again, in the authors' experience, it is unlikely to overtension the repair. In fact, research by Takahashi and colleagues[29] showed that overtensioning may "account for any plastic deformation of the

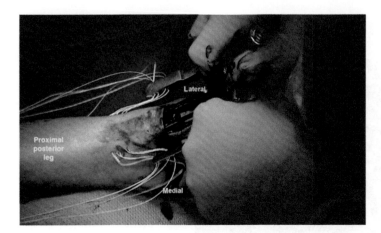

Fig. 6. Slide the jig distally out of the wound while managing the suture on each side of the tendon. Use a hemostat to gently deliver each loop of sutures from the wound. (*Adapted from* Liechti DJ, Moatshe G, Backus JD, et al. A Percutaneous Knotless Technique for Acute Achilles Tendon Ruptures. Arthrosc Tech 2018;7(2):e173; with permission.)

Achilles prior to its rupture and compensate for suture creep. It appears that the body may have inherent ability to compensate via sarcomere addition and subsequent tendon lengthening."

Some surgeons will choose to place a peritendinous suture at the tendon edges at the transverse incision. Closure of the paratenon with an absorbable suture is the authors' preference because this technique has been shown to strengthen the repair.[23,30,31]

COMPLICATIONS AND MANAGEMENT

An overview of pearls and pitfalls are presented in (Table 1). Failure to bury each calcaneal anchor into the tunnels can present as heel pain at the anchor sites. This complication is usually associated with edema around the anchor sites on MRI. The height of the anchor can be checked by backing out the anchor handle and placing a Freer elevator on the bony surface. The calcaneal bone is of sufficient quality to bury the anchor threads below the cortex.

Tendon elongation can be caused by several technical errors. Failure to precondition the sutures may lead to creep. Failure of the sutures to adequately obtain purchase in the proximal tendon will also lead to inadequate restoration of length. Clanton and colleagues[26] found that 80% of the total elongation occurred by the first 10 cycles of loading. The authors endorse aggressively preconditioning the sutures for this reason. Preconditioning will, in the authors'

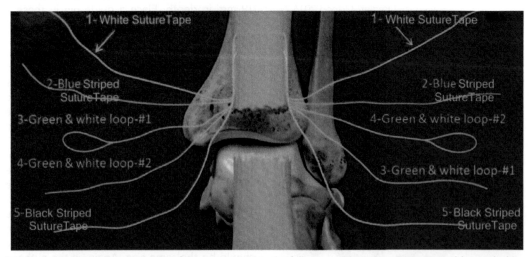

Fig. 7. Arrange the sutures outside of the wound bed in the following order: white SutureTape, blue and white–striped SutureTape, 1 green and white–striped suture with loop lateral, and 1 green and white–striped suture with loop medial, and most distally black and white–striped SutureTape. (This image provided courtesy of Arthrex®, Naples, Florida 2020.)

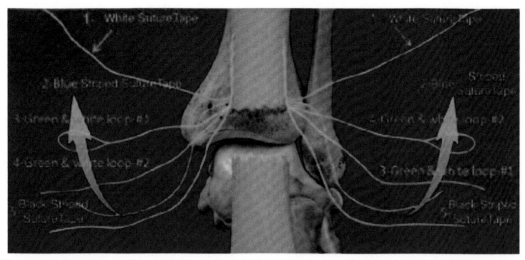

Fig. 8. Take the blue and white–striped SutureTape underneath; wrap it around the green and white sutures twice, and place it through the loop on each side. (This image provided courtesy of Arthrex®, Naples, Florida 2020.)

opinion, "minimize postoperative suture stretch and creep and decrease postoperative tendon lengthening."[25]

ADVANTAGES OF THE PERCUTANEOUS ACHILLES REPAIR SYSTEM AND ACHILLES MIDSUBSTANCE SpeedBridge

Histopathologic changes occur at the proximal and distal stumps of the tendon during the injury, including changes in collagen architecture, vascularity, and healing response.[32] Although most Achilles repair techniques pass

sutures directly through this compromised tendon, each of the techniques presented in this article avoid the affected tendon and, in theory, optimize the fixation.

POSTOPERATIVE CARE

Postoperatively, early active rehabilitation instructed by a physical therapist is crucial (Table 2). Immediately after surgery, the patient receives a splint and is non-weight-bearing. After 10 to 14 days, the splint is removed. The incision is typically healed at this point, and sutures can

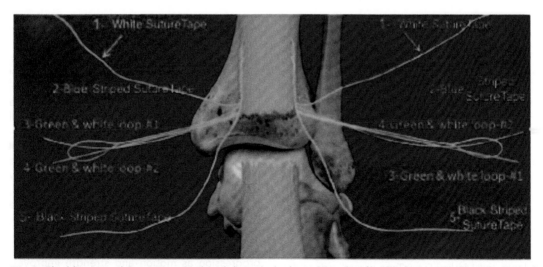

Fig. 9. The blue-striped SutureTape is placed through the loop on each side. (This image provided courtesy of Arthrex®, Naples, Florida 2020.)

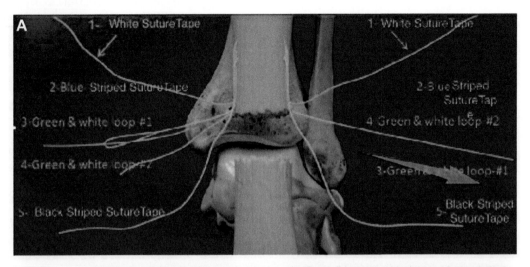

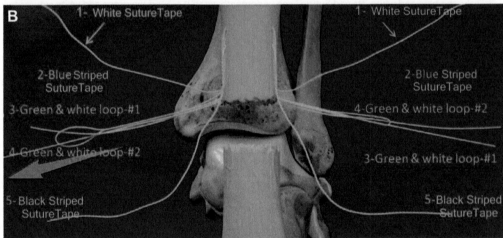

Fig. 10. (*A, B*) Pull on the nonlooped side of the green and white sutures on each side of the leg and remove the green and white sutures from the field. (This image provided courtesy of Arthrex®, Naples, Florida 2020.)

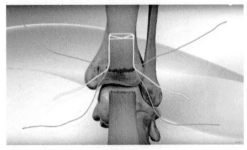

Fig. 11. The construct consists of 2 nonlocking SutureTapes and 1 locked SutureTape on each side of the tendon. (*Courtesy* of Arthrex, Naples, FL; with permission.)

be removed. The patient is transitioned to a walking boot with 4 felt wedges (Hapad, Bethel Park, PA, USA) placed under the heel, each with a maximum thickness of 7/16 in. At this time, the patient is allowed to begin transitioning to full weight-bearing over the next 4 weeks. In addition, therapist-guided active plantar and dorsal flexion up to 5° less than the contralateral ankle is started. One heel wedge is removed every week. At 7 weeks, the walking boot is removed, and the patient can start walking in a shoe. One or 2 wedges may be used in the shoe during the first 2 weeks if necessary for comfort. At 9 weeks, functional physiotherapy is started with gradual progression as motion and strength improves, but activities are restricted until 16 weeks because the risk of rerupture is high during this

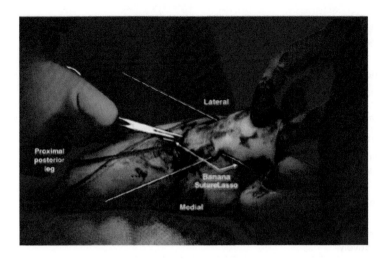

Fig. 12. A Banana SutureLasso is passed through each incision in a retrograde direction. This will emerge through the previous transverse incision. (This image provided courtesy of Arthrex®, Naples, Florida 2020.)

time. At 16 weeks, athletes can resume controlled practice with pain as a guide for limitations. Athletes are usually able to return to full participation 6 to 9 months postoperatively. However, full recovery may take up to 1 year.

OUTCOMES

Minimally invasive Achilles repair was developed in order to maintain the benefit of surgical repair with reduced rerupture rate and greater plantar flexion strength, while avoiding the soft tissue

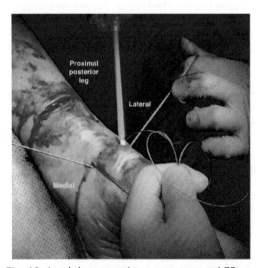

Fig. 13. Load the respective sutures onto a 4.75-mm BioComposite SwiveLock anchor and place them into the calcaneus tunnels. While turning the paddle so, be sure to pull axial traction. (This image provided courtesy of Arthrex®, Naples, Florida 2020.)

complications and morbidity associated with the standard open technique. Several large metaanalyses have shown improved clinical results and less wound problems and complication rates with minimally invasive techniques.

A metaanalysis by Grassi and colleagues[33] compared 182 patients treated with minimally invasive surgery and 176 treated with open repair and found a significantly decreased rate of overall complications, especially wound infection, and better patient-reported outcomes after minimally invasive surgery with no difference in rerupture rate or sural nerve injury. Another metaanalysis of 277 Achilles tendon repairs from randomized controlled trials by McMahon and colleagues[34] also showed no significant difference in complications (rerupture, tissue adhesion, deep infection, sural nerve injury, deep vein thrombosis) between minimally invasive and open repair, but a significantly reduced rate of superficial wound infection and 3 times greater patient satisfaction with minimally invasive approaches. A metaanalysis of 443 patients comparing Achillon to open repair found significantly increased rates of complications in the open group, but no significant differences in rerupture rate, sural nerve injury, return to sports, and AOFAS score following repair between the 2 groups.[21]

More literature has been published in recent years on the newer PARS method. A retrospective review of 101 PARS and 169 open cases by Hsu and colleagues[35] showed no significant differences in postoperative complications, but did show that a greater number of patients treated with the PARS were able to return to baseline physical activity by 5 months. A

Table 1
Pearls and pitfalls of the Achilles Midsubstance Speedbridge technique

Pearls	Pitfalls
Be familiar with the instrumentation	Incision too distal from the rupture
Palpate the Achilles tendon and locate the rupture before incision	Not placing the percutaneous Achilles Repair System jig proximal enough resulting in poor tendon capture with the sutures
Incision 1 cm proximal to the rupture	Sutures entangling poor suture management
Separate the Achilles tendon from the paratenon to enhance healing and protect the sural nerve	Undertensioning the repair using SwiveLocks
Passing and pulling the sutures in the right order to avoid entangling	Not inserting SwiveLocks completely into calcaneal tunnels
Immobilizing the ankle joint in a stirrup and posterior slab 1–2 wk postoperatively	

From Liechti DJ, Moatshe G, Backus JD, et al. A Percutaneous Knotless Technique for Acute Achilles Tendon Ruptures. Arthrosc Tech 2018;7(2):e176; with permission.

Table 2
The Achilles Midsubstance Speedbridge postoperative rehabilitation protocol

Time	Therapy
Weeks 1–2	Non-weight-bearing in a postoperative splint
Weeks 3	Walking boot with 4 heel wedges, start 4-wk weight-bearing progression, removal of 1 wedge per week, allowed to start active plantar flexion and dorsiflexion up to 5° to 10° short to neutral. Formal PT can start at this time for range of motion
Week 7	Wean from boot to shoe with 2 wedges, remove 1 wedge per week
Week 8	Start functional PT with sports progression
Week 12–16	Limit activities in athletes to practice. Risk of rerupture persists up to 4 mo
Week 16	Start controlled practice with pain as guide
Months 4.5–12	Athletes able to return to the full preinjury level of activity as symptoms allow

Abbreviation: PT, physical therapy.
From Liechti DJ, Moatshe G, Backus JD, et al. A Percutaneous Knotless Technique for Acute Achilles Tendon Ruptures. Arthrosc Tech 2018;7(2):e177; with permission.

biomechanical study comparing the PARS to open Krackow repair showed no significant difference in load and work to failure, but did show a higher initial linear stiffness for open repair, which could potentially reduce gap formation during postoperative rehabilitation.[36] Another biomechanical study showed that the PARS device demonstrated a higher load to failure compared with the Achillon device.[24] The failure mode of the PARS device was at the suture-tendon interface, which also has been reported as the failure mode with the Krackow suture.[23,26]

The clinical results of the newest minimally invasive knotless technique, the Achilles Midsubstance SpeedBridge, are primarily limited to case reports,[37] but the initial reports are promising and support early rehabilitation and early return to sports. A preliminary report of 34 patients showed no complications and satisfactory outcomes.[25] A cadaveric study compared open repair with 3 minimally invasive techniques (the PARS, Achillon, and SpeedBridge) and found that open repair had significantly less early elongation compared with the other techniques. However, there was no significant difference in the total number of cycles to failure between open and minimally invasive techniques.[26] Another biomechanical comparison of 3 techniques: open Krackow, the PARS, and the PARS modified with suture anchors into the calcaneus, showed the greatest ultimate load to failure with the suture anchor modification and a trend toward stronger repair with cyclical loading at all times points.[38] Also, a cadaveric study showed that an anchor augmented

Krackow suture was stronger biomechanically in Achilles ruptures with a short distal stump than Krackow suture alone.[39]

SUMMARY

Minimally invasive surgical repair of acute Achilles ruptures has proven to be a safe and reliable option in patients with higher physical demands. Compared with open repair, it can restore function and level of activity quickly with low complication rates. The technique has evolved over years, and the authors believe that the Achilles Midsubstance SpeedBridge offers the strongest construct and is the preferred method of fixation.

DISCLOSURE

The following is a complete list of disclosures for Dr T. Clanton as well as The Steadman Philippon Research Institute: (1) received royalties for any pharmaceutical, biomaterial, or orthopedic product or device: Arthrex, Inc, Stryker, Inc; (2) within the past 12 months, served on a speakers' bureau or have been paid an honorarium to present by any pharmaceutical, biomaterial, or orthopedic product or device company: Arthrex, Inc, Stryker, Inc; (3) received consultancy fees for any pharmaceutical, biomaterial, or orthopedic device and equipment company, or supplier: Arthrex, Inc, Stryker, Inc; (4) received research or institutional support as a principal investigator from any pharmaceutical, biomaterial, orthopedic device and equipment company, or supplier: Arthrex; (5) received royalties, financial or material support from publishers: None; (6) served as board member/committee appointment for a society: Committee member of Foot and Ankle International's Managerial Board; (7) The Steadman Philippon Research Institute has received financial support from the following: Arthrex, Ossur Americas, Siemens Medical Solutions USA, Smith & Nephew Endoscopy, Arthrex, Inc. There are no disclosures for Drs I.K. Stake, K. Bartush, or M.D. Jamieson.

REFERENCES

1. Lantto I, Heikkinen J, Flinkkila T, et al. Epidemiology of Achilles tendon ruptures: increasing incidence over a 33-year period. Scand J Med Sci Sports 2015;25(1):e133–8.

2. Huttunen TT, Kannus P, Rolf C, et al. Acute Achilles tendon ruptures: incidence of injury and surgery in Sweden between 2001 and 2012. Am J Sports Med 2014;42(10):2419–23.

3. Clayton RA, Court-Brown CM. The epidemiology of musculoskeletal tendinous and ligamentous injuries. Injury 2008;39(12):1338–44.

4. Raikin SM, Garras DN, Krapchev PV. Achilles tendon injuries in a United States population. Foot Ankle Int 2013;34(4):475–80.

5. Kadakia AR, Dekker RG 2nd, Ho BS. Acute Achilles tendon ruptures: an update on treatment. J Am Acad Orthop Surg 2017;25(1):23–31.

6. Willits K, Amendola A, Bryant D, et al. Operative versus nonoperative treatment of acute Achilles tendon ruptures: a multicenter randomized trial using accelerated functional rehabilitation. J Bone Joint Surg Am 2010;92(17):2767–75.

7. Nilsson-Helander K, Silbernagel KG, Thomee R, et al. Acute Achilles tendon rupture: a randomized, controlled study comparing surgical and nonsurgical treatments using validated outcome measures. Am J Sports Med 2010;38(11):2186–93.

8. Olsson N, Silbernagel KG, Eriksson BI, et al. Stable surgical repair with accelerated rehabilitation versus nonsurgical treatment for acute Achilles tendon ruptures: a randomized controlled study. Am J Sports Med 2013;41(12):2867–76.

9. Wilkins R, Bisson LJ. Operative versus nonoperative management of acute Achilles tendon ruptures: a quantitative systematic review of randomized controlled trials. Am J Sports Med 2012;40(9):2154–60.

10. Olsson N, Nilsson-Helander K, Karlsson J, et al. Major functional deficits persist 2 years after acute Achilles tendon rupture. Knee Surg Sports Traumatol Arthrosc 2011;19(8):1385–93.

11. Lantto I, Heikkinen J, Flinkkila T, et al. A prospective randomized trial comparing surgical and nonsurgical treatments of acute Achilles tendon ruptures. Am J Sports Med 2016;44(9):2406–14.

12. Krackow KA, Thomas SC, Jones LC. Ligament-tendon fixation: analysis of a new stitch and comparison with standard techniques. Orthopedics 1988;11(6):909–17.

13. Khan RJ, Fick D, Keogh A, et al. Treatment of acute Achilles tendon ruptures. A meta-analysis of randomized, controlled trials. J Bone Joint Surg Am 2005;87(10):2202–10.

14. Soroceanu A, Sidhwa F, Aarabi S, et al. Surgical versus nonsurgical treatment of acute Achilles tendon rupture: a meta-analysis of randomized trials. J Bone Joint Surg Am 2012;94(23):2136–43.

15. Ma GW, Griffith TG. Percutaneous repair of acute closed ruptured Achilles tendon: a new technique. Clin Orthop Relat Res 1977;(128):247–55.

16. Wong J, Barrass V, Maffulli N. Quantitative review of operative and nonoperative management of Achilles tendon ruptures. Am J Sports Med 2002;30(4):565–75.

17. Kakiuchi M. A combined open and percutaneous technique for repair of tendo Achillis. Comparison with open repair. J Bone Joint Surg Br 1995;77(1):60–3.

18. Elton JP, Bluman EM. Limited open Achilles tendon repair with modified ring forceps: technique tip. Foot Ankle Int 2010;31(10):914–5.

19. Keller A, Ortiz C, Wagner E, et al. Mini-open tenor-rhaphy of acute Achilles tendon ruptures: medium-term follow-up of 100 cases. Am J Sports Med 2014;42(3):731–6.

20. Assal M, Jung M, Stern R, et al. Limited open repair of Achilles tendon ruptures: a technique with a new instrument and findings of a prospective multi-center study. J Bone Joint Surg Am 2002;84(2):161–70.

21. Alcelik I, Saeed ZM, Haughton BA, et al. Achillon versus open surgery in acute Achilles tendon repair. Foot Ankle Surg 2018;24(5):427–34.

22. Calder JD, Saxby TS. Early, active rehabilitation following mini-open repair of Achilles tendon rupture: a prospective study. Br J Sports Med 2005;39(11):857–9.

23. Lee SJ, Sileo MJ, Kremenic IJ, et al. Cyclic loading of 3 Achilles tendon repairs simulating early postoperative forces. Am J Sports Med 2009;37(4):786–90.

24. Demetracopoulos CA, Gilbert SL, Young E, et al. Limited-open Achilles tendon repair using locking sutures versus nonlocking sutures: an in vitro model. Foot Ankle Int 2014;35(6):612–8.

25. McWilliam JR, Mackay G. The internal brace for midsubstance Achilles ruptures. Foot Ankle Int 2016;37(7):794–800.

26. Clanton TO, Haytmanek CT, Williams BT, et al. A biomechanical comparison of an open repair and 3 minimally invasive percutaneous Achilles tendon repair techniques during a simulated, progressive rehabilitation protocol. Am J Sports Med 2015;43(8):1957–64.

27. Liechti DJ, Moatshe G, Backus JD, et al. A percutaneous knotless technique for acute Achilles tendon ruptures. Arthrosc Tech 2018;7(2):e171–8.

28. Schipper O, Cohen B. The acute injury of the Achilles: surgical options (open treatment, and, minimally invasive surgery). Foot Ankle Clin 2017;22(4):689–714.

29. Takahashi M, Ward SR, Marchuk LL, et al. Asynchronous muscle and tendon adaptation after surgical tensioning procedures. J Bone Joint Surg Am 2010;92(3):664–74.

30. Shepard ME, Lindsey DP, Chou LB. Biomechanical testing of epitenon suture strength in Achilles tendon repairs. Foot Ankle Int 2007;28(10):1074–7.

31. Shepard ME, Lindsey DP, Chou LB. Biomechanical comparison of the simple running and cross-stitch epitenon sutures in Achilles tendon repairs. Foot Ankle Int 2008;29(5):513–7.

32. Maffulli N, Longo UG, Maffulli GD, et al. Marked pathological changes proximal and distal to the site of rupture in acute Achilles tendon ruptures. Knee Surg Sports Traumatol Arthrosc 2011;19(4):680–7.

33. Grassi A, Amendola A, Samuelsson K, et al. Minimally invasive versus open repair for acute Achilles tendon rupture: meta-analysis showing reduced complications, with similar outcomes, after minimally invasive surgery. J Bone Joint Surg Am 2018;100(22):1969–81.

34. McMahon SE, Smith TO, Hing CB. A meta-analysis of randomised controlled trials comparing conventional to minimally invasive approaches for repair of an Achilles tendon rupture. Foot Ankle Surg 2011;17(4):211–7.

35. Hsu AR, Jones CP, Cohen BE, et al. Clinical outcomes and complications of percutaneous Achilles repair system versus open technique for acute Achilles tendon ruptures. Foot Ankle Int 2015;36(11):1279–86.

36. Dekker RG, Qin C, Lawton C, et al. A biomechanical comparison of limited open versus Krackow repair for Achilles tendon rupture. Foot & Ankle Orthopaedics 2017;2(4):1–7. https://doi.org/10.1177/2473011417715431.

37. Byrne PA, Hopper GP, Wilson WT, et al. Knotless repair of Achilles tendon rupture in an elite athlete: return to competition in 18 weeks. J Foot Ankle Surg 2017;56(1):121–4.

38. Cottom JM, Baker JS, Richardson PE, et al. Evaluation of a new knotless suture anchor repair in acute Achilles tendon ruptures: a biomechanical comparison of three techniques. J Foot Ankle Surg 2017;56(3):423–7.

39. Boin MA, Dorweiler MA, McMellen CJ, et al. Suture-only repair versus suture anchor-augmented repair for Achilles tendon ruptures with a short distal stump: a biomechanical comparison. Orthop J Sports Med 2017;5(1). 2325967116678722.

Percutaneous Techniques in Orthopedic Foot and Ankle Surgery

Oliver N. Schipper, MD[a,*], Jonathan Day, MS[b],
Gabrielle S. Ray, BA[c], Anne Holly Johnson, MD[b]

KEYWORDS

- Minimally invasive • PECA • MICA • MIS bunion surgery • MIS bunionectomy
- MIS foot and ankle surgery

KEY POINTS

- There is a growing application for percutaneous techniques in orthopedic foot and ankle surgery.
- Many minimally invasive procedures, including percutaneous bunionectomy and lesser toe corrective surgery, result in good clinical and radiographic outcomes with minimal complications.
- As these procedures become more widely adopted, it is important to educate surgeons on proper technique and management.
- Although early results are promising, there is a need for large, long-term clinical studies to be conducted.

PERCUTANEOUS BUNIONECTOMY

Introduction and Background for Percutaneous Bunionectomy

Percutaneous correction of hallux valgus was first described by Vernois and colleagues[1] and Redfern and colleagues,[2] in 2011, when they developed a minimally invasive chevron and Akin (MICA) technique.[1,2] The advantages of this technique were to combine the benefits of percutaneous osteotomies while achieving rigid internal fixation for bony correction (Fig. 1). Although the literature has been limited, several important studies since then have investigated the efficacy and outcomes of this procedure.

In a recent retrospective comparative study by Lai and colleagues,[3] the investigators compared early clinical and radiographic outcomes at 2-year follow-up between MICA (n = 29) and open scarf/Akin osteotomies (n = 58) for bunion correction. They reported comparable clinical outcomes (American Orthopaedic Foot and Ankle Society [AOFAS] and 36-Item Short Form Health Survey) and radiographic correction of the 1-2 intermetatarsal angle (IMA), with significantly greater improvement in hallux valgus angle (HVA) in the percutaneous cohort compared with those that underwent scarf/Akin osteotomy. In addition, the percutaneous cohort demonstrated significantly less pain (visual analog scale [VAS]) and had no wound complications compared with 3 wound complications in the open cohort. In a similar, prospective randomized study performed by Lee and colleagues,[4] the investigators compared early clinical and radiographic outcomes between a cohort of 25 patients randomized to undergo MICA and 25 patients randomized to undergo scarf/Akin osteotomy. The investigators reported comparable AOFAS

---

[a] Anderson Orthopaedic Clinic, 2445 Army Navy Drive, Arlington, VA 22206, USA; [b] Hospital for Special Surgery, 535 East 70th Street, New York, NY 10021, USA; [c] Tufts University School of Medicine, 145 Harrison Avenue, Boston, MA, USA
* Corresponding author.
E-mail address: oschipper@andersonclinic.com

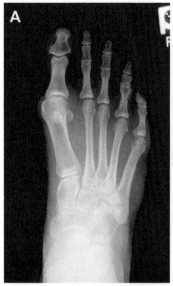
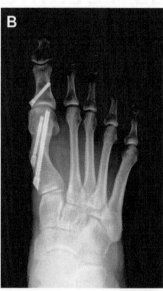
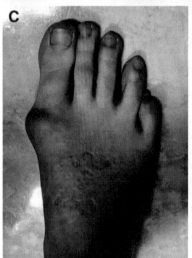
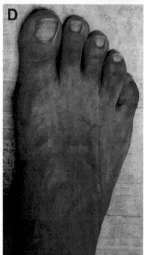

Fig. 1. (*A, B*) Preoperative and 4-month postoperative AP radiographs demonstrating hallux valgus correction with percutaneous bunionectomy. (*C, D*) Corresponding preoperative and 4-month postoperative clinical photos demonstrating good correction.

patient-reported outcomes as well as radiographic correction of both the HVA and IMA between the 2 cohorts at 6 months' follow-up. The MICA cohort demonstrated significantly less pain at 6 weeks' follow-up.

Surgical Technique for Percutaneous Bunionectomy
Preoperative planning

- Consider patient bone quality and any prior hardware in place.

Indications

- Mild to severe flexible hallux valgus deformities in which the 1-2 IMA is not greater than the width of the first metatarsal head.

- Revision of hallux valgus deformities

Contraindications

- Rigid hallux valgus deformities

Preparation and patient positioning

- The patient typically is positioned supine with the operative foot off of the bed distally and externally rotated slightly away from the body to facilitate anteroposterior (AP) and lateral fluoroscopy views of the forefoot with minimal adjustment of the mini C-arm.
- The operative leg is elevated on a bump or blankets.
- The nonoperative leg may be frog-legged proximally away from the field and taped.

- The mini C-arm typically is positioned to the right of the patient for right-handed surgeons and to the left of the patient for left-handed surgeons, although this may be altered based on surgeon preference.

PERCUTANEOUS DISTAL FIRST METATARSAL OSTEOTOMY WITH AKIN BUNIONECTOMY
Distal First Metatarsal Osteotomy

1. The procedure may be performed with or without a tourniquet.
   a. Use of tourniquet may increase the chance of bone necrosis so adequate irrigation is necessary.
   b. If no tourniquet is used, the patient may be placed in 10° to 20° of Trendelenburg to reduce bony bleeding during the case.
2. The first metatarsal is marked out using a skin marker and a guide wire is used to mark out the central axis on a lateral fluoroscopy view.
3. Using fluoroscopic guidance, a 3-mm to 5-mm mm medial, percutaneous, longitudinal incision is made at the metadiaphyseal junction of the medial first metatarsal (**Fig. 2**). A hemostat is used to bluntly dissect down to bone. Take care to avoid damaging the dorsomedial sensory nerve branch. A periosteal elevator is used to elevate soft tissue dorsally but not plantarly to avoid damaging the blood supply to the first metatarsal head.

4. (Optional) At this point, the surgeon may choose to use the 3.1-mm wedge burr to resect the first metatarsal head medial eminence (5000 rpm) with the advantage that the eminence is most prominent and stable prior to distal first metatarsal osteotomy. Alternatively, resection of the medial eminence may not be necessary after lateral translation of the metatarsal head and/or still may be performed after stable fixation of the osteotomy at the end of the procedure. In order to perform the medial eminence excision, the 3.1-mm wedge burr is inserted directly into the medial eminence using AP fluoroscopic guidance. The medial eminence (2 mm) then is resected with rotation of the hand plantar and dorsal. The surgeon should use copious irrigation with use of the burr to prevent thermal injury to the skin and bone. Bone debris may be expressed from the skin incision or removed with a large angiocatheter.
5. The 2.2-mm × 22-mm Shannon burr then is inserted (5000 rpm) under AP fluoroscopic guidance into the base of the medial first metatarsal head flare slightly more dorsal than plantar (one-third dorsal and two-third plantar). The burr is angled 10° plantarly and distally to reduce the risk of transfer metatarsalgia and prevent shortening of the first ray. Once the burr tip has reached the lateral cortex, an AP fluoroscopy view is obtained to confirm the trajectory of the burr (**Fig. 3**). The burr then is passed through the lateral cortex to create the apex of the chevron osteotomy.

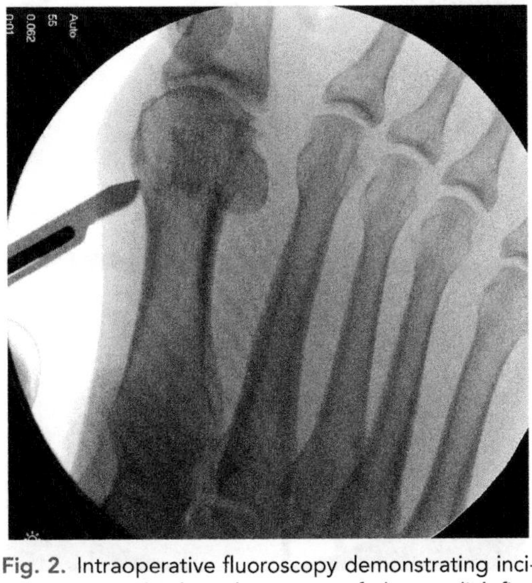

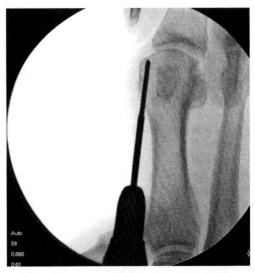

Fig. 2. Intraoperative fluoroscopy demonstrating incision at metadiaphyseal junction of the medial first metatarsal.

Fig. 3. Intraoperative fluoroscopy confirming trajectory of the burr and position at the lateral cortex.

Alternatively, a vertical transverse osteotomy may be performed. With larger shifts, the type of osteotomy becomes less relevant secondary to less bony contact.

6. For each limb of the osteotomy, the surgeon should envision the endpoint of the hand position prior to each cut. First complete the dorsal vertical limb of the short chevron osteotomy by rotating the hand plantar and slightly proximal, using the medial cortex osteotomy hole as the center of rotation (fulcrum). As the osteotomy is performed, the surgeon should gently oscillate the burr in and out to ensure that the far cortex is cut. Consider gentle irrigation of the incision and burr to prevent skin thermal injury.

7. Next, return the burr to the apex of the osteotomy. Complete the plantar limb of the chevron osteotomy by rotating the hand dorsal and slightly distally, using the medial cortex osteotomy hole as the center of rotation for the osteotomy. Keep the plantar limb of the chevron cut short to allow for easier rotational correction.

8. Ensure that the osteotomy is complete prior to attempting to shift head to prevent a small cortical bridge bone spike from limiting head translation.

9. Once the capital fragment is mobile, pull traction on the hallux and insert the thick end of the head-shifting tool through the same first metatarsal medial eminence incision and into the first metatarsal shaft.

10. Pull traction on the hallux and place a varus stress on the hallux to shift the first metatarsal head laterally relative to the shaft. Take care to maintain proper sagittal alignment and rotation of the head relative to the shaft with use of AP and lateral fluoroscopy views.

11. Fixation of the construct should include 2 screws, ideally 3.0 mm to 4.0 mm fully threaded cannulated screws. Beveled screws are preferable because they diminish the risk of hardware prominence. Although the size of the screw may vary depending on surgeon preference, the proper position of the screws is crucial to maintained stable fixation. The authors' preferred technique is to place two 4.0-mm fully threaded cannulated screws secondary to easier use of the 1.4-mm guide wire and greater stability of the construct. The first wire is inserted through the proximal medial cortex midaxially at the base of first metatarsal shaft, angling

approximately 1 cm lateral to the first metatarsal head. The guide wire must be placed through the proximal medial and the distal lateral first metatarsal shaft cortices prior to engaging the capital fragment for stability of the construct. Check AP and lateral fluoroscopy views to ensure that the trajectory of the wire is correct. Alternatively, the guide wire may be inserted after the amount of head shift is approximated initially with use of the head-shifting tool.

12. Obtain AP and lateral fluoroscopy views to check first metatarsal position and then drive the guide wire into the capital fragment after correction of IMA, distal metatarsal articular angle, and pronation.

13. Next insert a second guide wire is inserted just distal to the first through the medial proximal first metatarsal cortex and into the capital fragment. Check AP and lateral fluoroscopy views to confirm guide wire position (**Fig. 4**).

14. Each guide wire then is measured and overdrilled and then the screws placed. Typically 4-6mm are subtracted from the guidewire measurement to prevent hardware prominence.

15. AP, internal oblique, and lateral fluoroscopy views are checked to confirm that the screw heads are not prominent and that the screw tips are not within the first metatarsophalangeal joint (MTPJ) (**Fig. 5**).

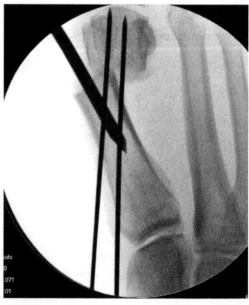

Fig. 4. Intraoperative fluoroscopy confirming guide wire positioning.

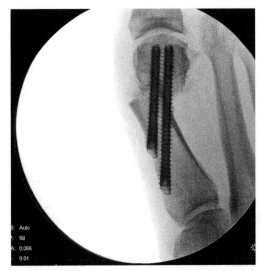

Fig. 5. Intraoperative fluoroscopy demonstrating that the screw tips are not within the first MTPJ.

16. Finally, the medial spike of first metatarsal shaft bone is excised using a Shannon burr through 1 of the existing incisions (typically the distal screw insertion incision). The medial spike is cut from plantar to dorsal to avoid damaging the dorsomedial sensory nerve branch. The free bone fragment either may be removed with a hemostat or pushed into the osteotomy site as bone graft.
17. If a medial eminence resection was not performed at the beginning of the case; a Shannon burr or wedge burr may be used to complete the resection at this point.
18. (Optional) For severe deformities, a lateral release of the lateral phalangeosesamoid ligament, lateral metatarsosesamoid ligament, and/or adductor hallucis tendon may be performed percutaneously through a dorsal lateral first MTPJ incision with use of a beaver blade and AP fluoroscopic guidance. Avoid cutting the lateral collateral ligament.

Akin Osteotomy

1. An Akin osteotomy may be performed if interphalangeous deformity is noted after the chevron or if further hallux valgus deformity corrected is desired. Under fluoroscopic guidance, the position of the ostetomy is marked at the metadiaphyseal margin of the medial proximal phalanx.
2. The 2-mm × 12-mm Shannon burr is inserted midaxially and angled retrograde

to while preserving the lateral cortex. Care is taken to avoid MTPJ (Fig. 6).
3. The dorsal limb is completed while holding the hallux interphalangeal joint dorsiflexed to prevent damage to the extensor hallucis longus tendon.
4. The plantar limb is completed with the hallux interphalangeal joint plantarflexed to prevent damage to the flexor hallucis longus tendon.
5. The hallux is placed in varus and greensticked, correcting any remaining valgus deformity. A wire then is placed percutaneously from the medial base of the hallux proximal phalanx across the Akin osteotomy site and through the distal lateral cortex. The position is checked on AP and lateral fluoroscopy views. The wire then is measured and overdrilled, and then a screw, typically 3.0 mm, is placed (Fig. 7).
6. The incisions are closed with a single suture or adhesive strips.
7. The incisions are dressed with a nonadherent layer and 4-in × 4-in gauze.
8. Gauze strips moistened with normal saline are placed in each of the web spaces and wrapped around the medial forefoot to maintain a varus stress.
9. A 2-in kling bandage then is wrapped around each toe sequentially from medial to lateral with a slight varus stress to maintain hallux valgus correction.
10. The cling is overwrapped with an ACE wrap.

Postoperative Care

- The dressing is left in place for 2 weeks and then a new dressing or soft toe splint is placed for another 2 weeks at the first postoperative visit.

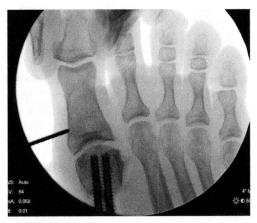

Fig. 6. Intraoperative fluoroscopy confirming the burr is not in the MTPJ.

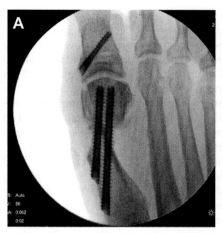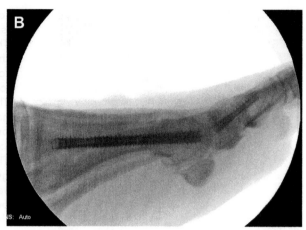

Fig. 7. (*A, B*) Final AP and lateral fluoroscopic views showing proper placement of PECA screw.

- Weight bearing as tolerated is allowed in a heel-bearing or flat postoperative shoe for the first 4 weeks to 6 weeks postoperatively. The patient then is transitioned to a supportive shoe as tolerated.
- A soft forefoot compression sleeve may be applied at 4 weeks postoperatively to assist with edema reduction.
- Physical therapy is offered after the wounds have healed.

Complications and Management

- Infection
  - Irrigation and débridement are recommended for deep infections with removal of hardware.
- Nonunion
  - Full radiographic bony union across the osteotomy may take 3 months to 6 months. In patients with persistent pain or evidence of screw breakage, a nonunion may be present. CT scan may be considered. Revision with compression plate and screws is recommended when present.
- Iatrogenic or postoperative fracture
  - Caution should be used in elderly patients with osteoporosis and patients with poor bone quality. Fracture may be managed with plate and screw fixation.
    - Consider using a lower burr speed in patients with poor bone quality.
    - Consider heel weight bearing for 6 weeks postoperatively for patients with poor bone quality.
- Screw prominence

  - A screw head may be left prominent over medial base of the first metatarsal or the tip of a screw may be left intra-articular.
    - Always check lateral and oblique fluoroscopy views to ensure that the screw tips are not intra-articular.
    - Consider taking off 2 mm to 4 mm from measured guide wire length for first metatarsal osteotomy and 2 mm off for Akin osteotomy.
- First metatarsal shortening
  - Always angle distally (and plantarly if performing chevron osteotomy) to prevent relative shortening of the 1st metatarsal.
- Skin thermal burn
  - Recommend avoidance of tourniquet and irrigation of the burr to prevent thermal injury.

PERCUTANEOUS LESSER TOE CORRECTION

Introduction and Background for Percutaneous Lesser Toe Correction

Percutaneous lesser toe corrections techniques offer a fast alternative to open procedures and employ a combination of bone and soft tissue procedures. Advantages include reduced risk of scar tissue formation and contractures and vascular and wound complications.

Surgical Technique for Percutaneous Lesser Toe Correction
Preoperative planning

- Consider patient bone quality, flexibility of deformity, and type of deformity.

Indications

- Any lesser toe deformity, flexible or rigid (Figs. 8 and 9)
- Any lesser toe interphalangeal joint instability or arthritis

Contraindications

- Infection of lesser toe

Preparation and patient positioning

- The patient typically is positioned supine with the operative foot off of the bed distally and a bump under the hip on the operative side.
- The operative leg is elevated on a bump or blankets.
- The nonoperative leg may be frog-legged proximally away from the field and taped.
- The mini C-arm typically is positioned to the right of the patient for right-handed surgeons and to the left of the patient for left-handed surgeons, although this may be altered based on surgeon preference.

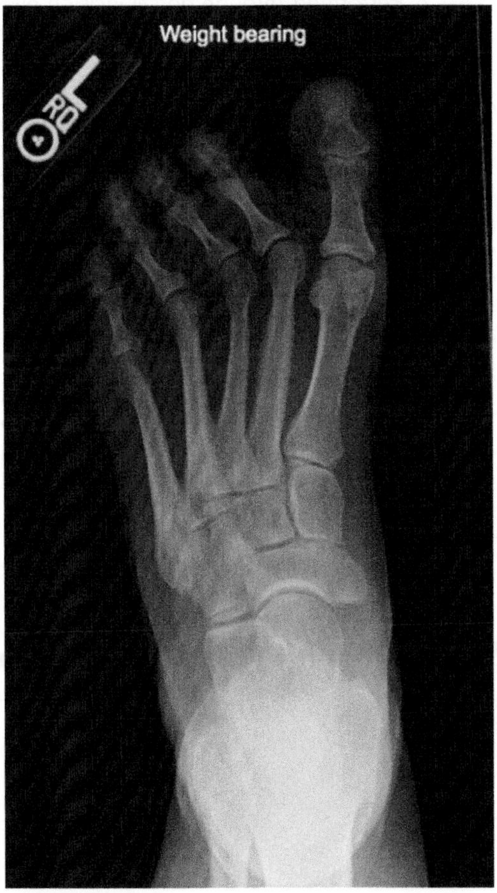

Extensor Digitorum Longus and Extensor Digitorum Brevis Tenotomies

- Performed where the 2 tendons are separated at the level of the dorsal MTPJ.
  - Fibroaponeurotic expansion of the extensor digitorum longus tendon prevents proximal retraction of the tendon.
- Used to correct MTPJ cock-up deformity (MTPJ dorsiflexion).
- Plantarflexion of MTPJ used to confirm complete tendon release.

Dorsal Metatarsophalangeal Joint Capsule Release

- Performed at level of MTPJ if extensor tenotomy insufficient or subluxation/dislocation of MTPJ.
- Used to correct MTPJ cock-up deformity (MTPJ dorsiflexion).
- Traction used to distract joint and tension capsule for sharp release using a #15 blade or beaver blade.

Weight bearing

Fig. 8. Weight-bearing AP radiograph of left foot preoperatively demonstrating significant deformity in second through fourth lesser toes.

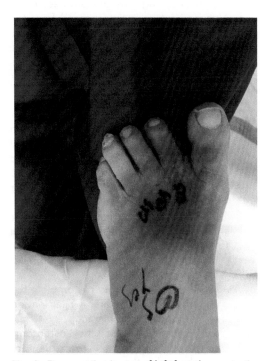

Fig. 9. Preoperative image of left foot demonstrating significant deformity in second through fourth lesser toes.

Flexor Digitorum Brevis Tenotomy

- Performed at level of medial or lateral proximal interphalangeal joint using a beaver blade with the proximal interphalangeal joint plantarflexed to protect the underlying neurovascular bundle.
- Used to correct rigid or flexible proximal interphalangeal joint plantarflexion deformity.
- Incision is made just proximal to the medial or lateral proximal interphalangeal joint using a beaver blade. Blade then is used to release the proximal interphalangeal joint plantar capsule. The flexor digitorum brevis slips then are sharply released off of the insertion at the base of the middle phalanx.

Flexor Digitorum Longus Tenotomy

- Performed at level of distal interphalangeal joint using a beaver blade via a plantar approach with simultaneous dorsiflexion of the distal interphalangeal joint.
- Used to correct flexible distal interphalangeal joint plantarflexion deformity.

Extra-Articular Proximal Phalanx Osteotomy

- Used to correct varus, valgus, and/or cock-up MTPJ deformities.
- Performed at the proximal metadiaphyseal region of the proximal phalanx.
- Plantar closing wedge osteotomy
  - The authors' preference is to perform osteotomy from medial or lateral (depending on surgeon hand dominance) to the metadiaphysis to facilitate use of AP fluoroscopy for guidance and avoid the flexor tendons.
    1. The 2-mm × 8-mm Shannon burr (4000 rpm) is inserted from medial or lateral just plantar to the dorsal cortex of the proximal phalanx and bicortical.
    2. The hand is rotated to complete the osteotomy plantarly while leaving the dorsal cortex intact.
    3. Plantarflexion of the osteotomy is attempted. If unable to plantarflex the osteotomy, continue to feather the remaining dorsal cortex using the 2-mm × 8-mm

Shannon burr until plantarflexion of the osteotomy is possible.
  - Alternatively, the osteotomy may be performed through a plantar approach at the proximal metadiaphyseal region of the proximal phalanx.
    1. The 2-mm × 8-mm Shannon burr (4000 rpm) is inserted around the flexor tendons and then through the plantar cortex.
    2. The burr is stopped at the dorsal cortex.
    3. The hand is rotated medially and laterally to complete the osteotomy while leaving the dorsal cortex intact.
    4. Plantarflexion of the osteotomy is attempted. If unable to plantarflex the osteotomy, ensure that the medial and lateral cortices have been completely osteotomized with the burr.
- Akinette osteotomy
  - Performed through dorsal incision over the proximal metadiaphyseal region of the proximal phalanx.
  - The 2-mm × 8-mm Shannon burr is inserted from dorsal to plantar through the proximal phalanx and then the osteotomy is completed medially to correct a valgus deformity leaving the lateral cortex intact, or laterally to correct a varus deformity, leaving the medial cortex intact (**Figs. 10 and 11**).

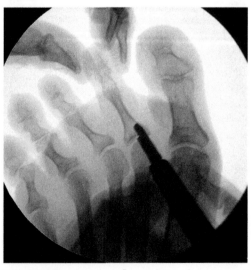

Fig. 10. Intraoperative fluoroscopy demonstrating starting location of burr for akinette osteotomy in correction of second toe deformity.

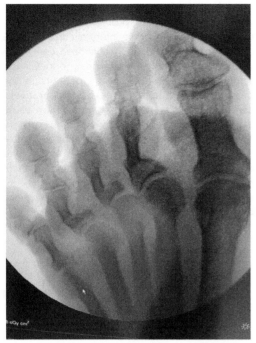

Fig. 11. Intraoperative fluoroscopy demonstrating completed akinette osteotomies of second through fourth toes.

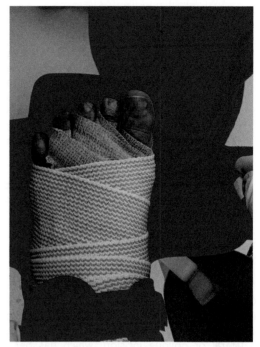

Fig. 12. Postoperative dressing applied strapping of the second through fourth toes in the desired position for healing.

○ Closure of the osteotomy is attempted. If unable to close down the osteotomy, continue to feather the remaining cortex using the 2-mm × 8-mm Shannon burr until closure of the osteotomy is possible.

- The osteotomies, described previously, may be combined to correct deformities in 2 planes.
  ○ For example, for a cock-up/varus second toe deformity with crossover the hallux, a plantar-lateral closing osteotomy of the proximal phalanx may be performed using the 2-mm × 8-mm Shannon burr (4000 rpm) to correct the deformity.
- The postoperative dressing must include strapping of the toe in the desired position for healing (Fig. 12). At 2 weeks, the patient is transitioned to a removable toe splint for another 3 weeks.

Extra-Articular Middle Phalanx Osteotomy

- Used to correct lesser toe proximal interphalangeal joint plantarflexion deformity
- Performed through dorsal incision over the diaphysis of the middle phalanx
- The 2-mm × 8-mm Shannon burr (4000 rpms) is inserted from dorsal to

plantar through the middle phalanx and stopped at the plantar cortex, leaving the plantar cortex intact.
- The burr is used to sweep medially and laterally to complete the osteotomy.
- The osteotomy then is closed down manually with dorsiflexion of the distal interphalangeal joint and a Steri-Strip is placed to hold the distal and proximal interphalangeal joints in a dorsiflexed position in order to allow the osteotomy to heal in a dorsiflexed position.
- The osteotomy is maintained in a dorsiflexed position for a total of 5 weeks postoperatively with Steri-Strips.

Complications and Management

- Infection
  ○ Oral antibiotics are recommended for superficial infections. Irrigation and débridement are recommended for deep infections.
- Nonunion
  ○ Full radiographic bony union across the osteotomy may take 3 months to 6 months. In patients with persistent pain, a nonunion may be present. CT scan may be considered. Revision with

Kirschner (K)-wire is recommended when present.

- Malunion
  - The initial postoperative dressing is important to maintain lesser toe deformity corrects given no hardware typically is used. The investigators recommend strapping the toes with a soft dressing, tape, or a removable toe splint for the first 5 weeks postoperatively.
- Skin thermal burn
  - Recommend avoidance of tourniquet and irrigation of the burr to prevent thermal injury.

PERCUTANEOUS CALCANEAL OSTEOTOMY

Introduction and Background for Percutaneous Calcaneal Osteotomy

Open calcaneal osteotomy often has been required in the surgical correction of hindfoot deformities. Traditional open techniques involve a lateral or oblique incision, which has been associated with neurovascular injury and wound healing issues, ranging from limited delay to skin necrosis and deep bone infection.[5–7] Complication rates of 5% to 28% have been reported in the literature.[6,7] Minimally invasive approaches employing percutaneous techniques have gained popularity in an effort to combat such high complication rates. In the past decade, there has been an evolution of such techniques aimed at minimizing soft tissue destruction and complications. Initially, DiDomenico and colleagues[8] described a percutaneous osteotomy using a Gigli saw inserted into a subperiosteal tunnel that looped up and over the calcaneus via 4 stab incisions, which resulted in no neurovascular damage in a cadaveric study of 20 limbs. A variant of this procedure later was described in which a suture was passed through a subperiosteal tunnel under arthroscopic guidance before shuttling a Gigli saw along the track.[9] Outcomes were reported on 25 patients without a single vascular injury, albeit 1 had persistent numbness in the sural nerve distribution.[9] More recently, a technique for percutaneous osteotomy has been described using a modification of the Shannon burr.[1]

A recent study of 122 patients compared results of calcaneal osteotomy for hindfoot realignment using the traditional open incision versus percutaneous technique with the Shannon burr.[7] Wound healing issues were observed in 15.5% of patients using the open approach, with two-thirds of these patients requiring wound débridement. Comparatively, there were no wound healing problems in the percutaneous group. Sural nerve injury occurred in 14% of patients with the open approach compared with only 6% in the percutaneous group. Clinical symptoms had resolved in all patients in the percutaneous group by 4 weeks postoperatively. Length of hospitalization also was shown to be significantly shorter in the percutaneous group.[7] This study concluded that percutaneous calcaneal osteotomy had excellent results and encouraged this procedure as a standard technique, especially for patients with high risk for wound healing complications, including diabetics and smokers.

Surgical Technique for Percutaneous Calcaneal Osteotomy

Preoperative planning

- Obtain dorsoplantar, lateral, and long hindfoot radiographs while weight bearing.

Indications

- Cavovarus or planovalgus foot deformity driven by malaligned calcaneus with an intact subtalar joint
- Failed nonoperative management with corrective foot orthoses

Contraindications

- Preexisting subtalar arthritis (relative contraindication)

Preparation and patient positioning

- The patient is positioned either lateral or supine, depending on concurrent procedures, with the limb available for manipulation for fluoroscopic guidance.
- The heel hangs off the end of the table perpendicular to or resting on the mini C-arm, which typically is positioned to the right of the patient if the surgeon is right-hand dominant (and on the left if left-hand dominant).

Percutaneous Calcaneal Osteotomy

- Using an elevator or other tool, the proposed position of the osteotomy is traced out on the lateral tuber using fluoroscopic guidance. The starting point for the burr in the center of the calcaneal tuber is also marked (Fig. 13).
- A 5-mm to 10-mm skin incision then is made at the center marked position. A

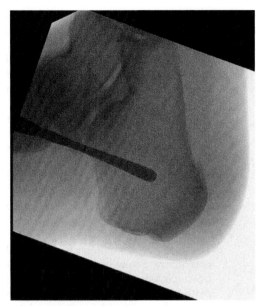

Fig. 13. Using fluoroscopic guidance, lateral calcaneal radiograph demonstrates a probe used to indicate the planned incision location of the posterior calcaneal osteotomy site.

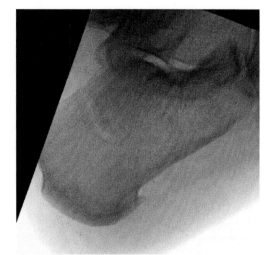

Fig. 14. Intraoperative fluoroscopy demonstrating dorsal chevron osteotomy.

hemostat is used to spread down to bone. Using the hemostat tines as retractors, the 3-mm × 30-mm Shannon burr is advanced into the calcaneal tuber at 6000 rpm. Fluoroscopy confirms that the burr is in the correct position at the center of the proposed osteotomy.

- The calcaneus is cut in 4 quadrants (superior lateral, superior medial, inferior lateral, and inferior lateral) using the center as the fulcrum to avoid placing too much torque on the burr, regardless of the shape of the osteotomy.
- Care should be taken to avoid burning both the skin and the bone by using copious cooling irrigation.
- Fluoroscopy should be checked periodically during the osteotomy to ensure that the burr trajectory is appropriate (Figs. 14 and 15).
- Once all 4 quadrants have been cut (Fig. 16), the calcaneus compresses across the osteotomy site and fluid exude from the incision.
- An elevator then may be placed inside the lateral cortex of the calcaneus and used to lever the tuber in the desired direction to correct either the valgus or varus malalignment.
- Guide wires are placed across the osteotomy and then screws are placed

to secure the osteotomy according to surgeon preference (Fig. 17).
- The lateral wound should be copiously irrigated to remove any bone paste, and then the skin closed with a nylon suture.

Postoperative Care

- Dressings and postoperative immobilization typically depend on concurrent procedures performed.
- Six weeks of non–weight bearing should allow for adequate healing of the calcaneal osteotomy.
- Physical therapy and further postoperative care depend on concurrent procedures performed.

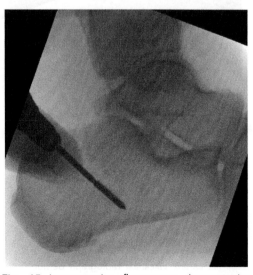

Fig. 15. Intraoperative fluoroscopy demonstrating plantar chevron osteotomy with burr.

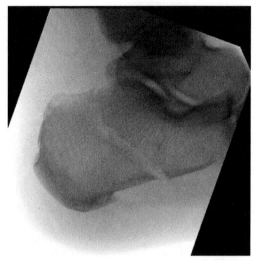

Fig. 16. Intraoperative fluoroscopy demonstrating completed dorsal and plantar chevron osteotomy.

Complications and Management

- Infection
  - Superficial infections may be treated with oral antibiotics, whereas deep infections may necessitate irrigation and débridement.
- Sural nerve injury
  - This is an iatrogenic complication that has been cited to occur in 5% to 28% of cases.[5,10] It can result in temporary or permanent irritation along the

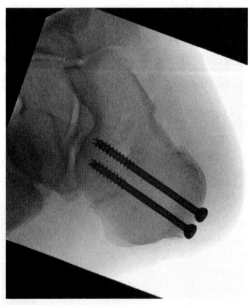

Fig. 17. Lateral calcaneal radiograph demonstrating stabilized osteotomy with 2 cannulated screws placed percutaneously.

course of sural nerve at the heel with neuroma formation and distal dysesthesia.
  - Gutteck and colleagues[7] found sural nerve injury occurred in 14% of patients with the open approach versus 6% in the percutaneous group.
  - By ensuring that the soft tissue is protected from the cutting tip of the burr upon entry into the bone, this complication risk is mitigated.
- Over-correction or under-correction of deformity
  - This may necessitate either repeated procedure or persistent malalignment.
- Painful hardware
  - This is relatively common for calcaneal osteotomy. Screw heads placed in the posteroinferior tuberosity or a lateral plate for a translational osteotomy are potential sources of hardware-related pain.
  - This can be treated by removal of hardware.
- Nonunion
  - Full radiographic bony union across the osteotomy may take 3 months to 6 months. In patients with persistent pain, a nonunion may be present. CT scan may be considered. Revision with compression plate and/or screws is recommended when present.
- Skin thermal burn
  - Recommend avoidance of tourniquet and irrigation of the burr to prevent thermal injury

PERCUTANEOUS BUNIONETTE OSTEOTOMY

Introduction and Background for Percutaneous Lateral Fifth Metatarsal Head Ostectomy and Fifth Distal Minimally Invasive Metatarsal Osteotomy

Minimally invasive techniques for management of fifth metatarsalgia and bunionette deformities have been developed to reduce pain and stiffness. Weil osteotomy is a well-documented technique for metatarsalgia but has a high incidence of floating toe.[11,12] Although early outcomes are promising, limited literature is available for distal metatarsal minimally invasive osteotomy secondary to the relatively recent introduction of the technique. In a case series of 30 patients who underwent distal metatarsal minimally invasive osteotomy for lesser metatarsalgia, the average Manchester-Oxford Foot Questionnaire (MOxFQ) score was excellent and the VAS improved by 3.5.[13] Two patients worsened after the procedure with regard to VAS and 4 complications were reported, including nonunion, malunion, transfer metatarsalgia, and heterotopic ossification. In a separate case series of 21 patients who underwent fifth distal metatarsal minimally invasive osteotomy for bunionette deformity, there was significant improvement in MOxFQ score and VAS.[14] There were no wound or nerve complications, but 1 patient required a dorsal cheilectomy for symptomatic dorsolateral callus formation at the osteotomy site.

Surgical Technique for Percutaneous Lateral Fifth Metatarsal Head Ostectomy and Fifth Distal Minimally Invasive Metatarsal Osteotomy
Preoperative planning

- Consider patient bone quality and any prior hardware in place.

Indications

- Type 1 bunionette deformity
- Type 2 bunionette deformity with IMA less than 12°
- Type 3 bunionette deformity with IMA less than 12°
- Fifth metatarsalgia

Contraindications

- Type 2 bunionette deformity with IMA greater than 12°
- Type 3 bunionette deformity with IMA greater than 12°

Preparation and patient positioning

- The patient typically is positioned supine with the operative foot off of the bed distally and a bump under the hip on the operative side.
- The operative leg is elevated on a bump or blankets.
- The nonoperative leg may be frog-legged proximally away from the field and taped.
- The mini C-arm typically is positioned to the right of the patient for right-handed surgeons and to the left of the patient for left-handed surgeons, although this may be altered based on surgeon preference.

Type 1 Bunionette Deformity

1. A small 2-mm to 3-mm incision is made over the dorsolateral fifth metatarsal distal

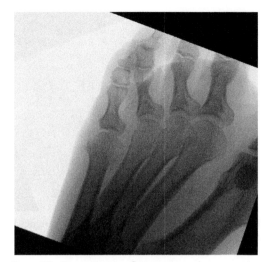

Fig. 18. Preoperative fluoroscopy demonstrating prominence of the bunionette deformity.

metaphyseal region approximately 1 cm from the lateral fifth metatarsal head (Fig. 18).
2. An elevator then is used to create a working space over the lateral fifth metatarsal head.
3. The 3.1-mm wedge burr is inserted into the lateral fifth metatarsal head under AP fluoroscopy imaging (Fig. 19).
4. The lateral fifth metatarsal head then is shaved down using a sweeping motion plantarly and dorsally until the lateral fifth metatarsal head is no longer prominent clinically and on AP fluoroscopy views (Fig. 20).
5. The incision then is irrigated with normal saline through an angiocatheter to remove any bone debris.

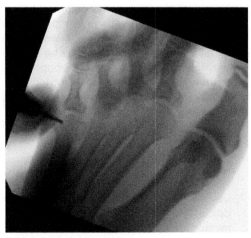

Fig. 19. Intraoperative fluoroscopy confirms proper insertion of the wedge burr.

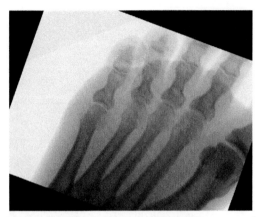

Fig. 20. Final AP fluoroscopic view confirms removal of bunionette.

6. A Steri-Strip is used to close the incision followed by a soft dressing.

Type 2 and Type 3 Bunionette Deformity

1. A small 2-mm to 3-mm incision is made over the dorsolateral fifth metatarsal distal metaphyseal region.
2. An elevator then is used to create as working space over the lateral fifth metatarsal head.
3. The 3.1-mm wedge burr is inserted into the lateral fifth metatarsal head under AP fluoroscopy imaging.
4. The lateral fifth metatarsal head then is shaved down using a sweeping motion plantarly and dorsally until the lateral fifth metatarsal head no longer is prominent clinically and on AP fluoroscopy views.
5. The surgeon then stands at the end of the foot. For a right foot, a separate dorsomedial incision is made at the distal metaphyseal region of the fifth metatarsal, whereas for a left foot, the same dorsolateral incision for lateral fifth metatarsal head ostectomy may be used in the right-handed surgeon. The opposite is performed for the left-handed surgeon.
6. The 2-mm × 12-mm burr then is introduced through the incision and placed at 45° angling plantar and retrograde at the distal fifth metatarsal metaphysis just outside of the fifth MTPJ capsule with use of lateral and slight oblique fluoroscopy views of the forefoot.
7. Using a sweeping motion of the hand from dorsal to plantar, the distal fifth metaphyseal osteotomy is completed and checked under lateral and slight oblique fluoroscopy views of the forefoot. The fifth

metatarsal head often shifts medial relative to the shaft secondary to soft tissue tension but also may be manually shifted medially. No fixation is necessary.
8. The remaining lateral fifth metatarsal shaft cortical spike may then be shaved down with a 3.1-mm wedge burr under AP fluoroscopy views of the forefoot.
9. The incision or incisions then are irrigated with normal saline through an angiocatheter to remove any bone debris.
10. A Steri-Strip is used to close the incision/s followed by a soft dressing.

Fifth Metatarsalgia

1. The surgeon stands at the end of the foot. For a right foot, a dorsomedial incision is made at the distal metaphyseal region of the fifth metatarsal, whereas for a left foot, a dorsolateral incision is made in the right-handed surgeon. The opposite is performed for the left-handed surgeon.
2. The 2-mm × 12-mm Shannon burr then is introduced through the incision and placed at 45° angling plantar and retrograde at the distal fifth metatarsal metaphysis just outside of the fifth MTPJ capsule with use of lateral and slight oblique fluoroscopy views of the forefoot (Fig. 21).
3. Using a sweeping motion of the hand from dorsal to plantar, the distal fifth metaphyseal osteotomy is completed and checked under lateral and slight oblique fluoroscopy views of the forefoot (Fig. 22). The fifth metatarsal head is allowed to shorten and elevate by 2 mm (width of the burr). No fixation is necessary.

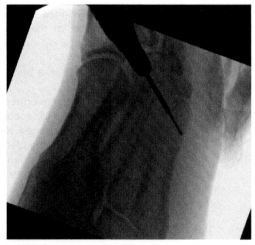

Fig. 21. Lateral fluoroscopic view demonstrates proper position and trajectory of the burr.

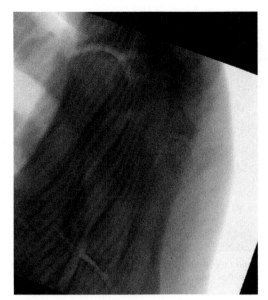

Fig. 22. Lateral fluoroscopic view confirms complete removal of the distal fifth metaphyseal prominence.

4. The incision then is irrigated with normal saline through an angiocatheter to remove any bone debris.
5. A Steri-Strip is used to close the incision/s followed by a soft dressing.

Postoperative Care

- The dressing is removed at 2 weeks postoperatively. The fifth toe may be taped for an additional 2 weeks for a type 2 or type 3 bunionette deformity in order to maintain correction.
- Weight bearing as tolerated is allowed in a flat postoperative shoe for the first 4 weeks postoperatively. The patient then is transitioned to a supportive shoe as tolerated.
- Activity may be increased as pain improves.

Complications and Management

- Infection
  - Irrigation and débridement are recommended for deep infections.
- Nonunion
  - Full radiographic bony union across the osteotomy may take 3 months to 6 months. In patients with persistent pain, a nonunion may be present. CT scan may be considered. Revision with compression plate and/or screws is recommended when present.
- Skin thermal burn

  - Recommend avoidance of tourniquet and irrigation of the burr to prevent thermal injury.

PERCUTANEOUS CHEILECTOMY
Introduction and Background for Percutaneous Cheilectomy

Similar to open cheilectomy, minimally invasive percutaneous cheilectomy is indicated for removal of the dorsal osteophyte and distal third of the metatarsal head to relieve pain and stiffness in patients with mild to moderate hallux rigidus.[15] Although studies have been limited, a recent case series performed by Teoh and colleagues[16] demonstrated that at an average follow-up of 50 months, patients treated with minimally invasive dorsal cheilectomy (MIDC) achieved significant improvement in the MOxFQ and VAS pain scores. The investigators concluded that MIDC is a safe technique with minimal complications similar to open cheilectomy. They reported 7 cases of first MTPJ arthrodesis, 4 repeat cheilectomies, 2 wound infections, and 2 cases of permanent numbness out of a cohort of 98 feet.[16] Another cases series comparing a cohort of 22 patients treated with MIDC with median 11 months' follow-up to a matched cohort of 25 patients treated with open cheilectomy with median 17 months' follow-up demonstrated that both groups had statistically significant improvement in MOxFQ.[17] The investigators reported 3 cases of first MTPJ arthrodesis in the open group versus none in the percutaneous cheilectomy group. Patient satisfaction as well as return to normal function and footwear have been shown to be similar between percutaneous cheilectomy and open cheilectomy.[18,19] In summary, early results of this new technique are encouraging, although larger, prospective comparative trials to identify a benefit over open cheilectomy have yet to be conducted.

Surgical Technique for Percutaneous Cheilectomy
Preoperative planning

- Obtain standing, weight-bearing plain radiographs of the foot in AP and lateral views to evaluate severity of articular degeneration (**Fig. 23**).

Indications

- Mild to moderate hallux rigidus that has failed trial of nonoperative management
- Presence of dorsal osteophyte causing impingement pain with dorsiflexion of

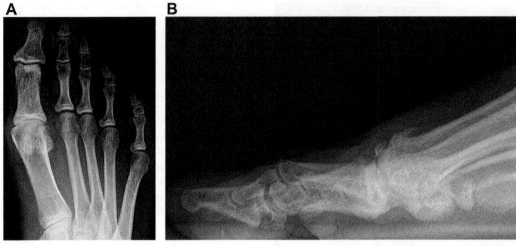

Fig. 23. Preoperative weight bearing (*A*) AP and (*B*) lateral plain radiographs demonstrating first metaphalangeal joint space narrowing and dorsal osteophyte in a patient with hallux rigidus.

the MTP or pressure from shoe wear on the prominent osteophyte

Contraindications

- Advanced articular surface osteoarthritis as shown clinically by a positive grind test[20]
- Pain with midrange motion or plantar pain suggesting inferior sesamoid degeneration
- Night pain or pain that occurs at rest
- Absence of dorsal osteophyte
- Any sign of infection

Preparation and patient positioning

- Patients may be discharged during the same day of surgery.
- The patient is positioned supine, with the limb free to allow for dorsoplantar rotation and lateral fluoroscopy.
- The heel hangs off the end of the table perpendicular to the mini C-arm, which is always positioned to the right of the patient regardless of which foot is being operated on.[21]

Percutaneous Cheilectomy

1. Use of a tourniquet generally is not required because the restriction of blood flow may promote thermal injury and prevent the cooling of the surgical site.
2. A longitudinal incision measuring 3 mm to 5 mm is made over the dorsomedial aspect of the first metatarsal, approximately 1 cm proximal to the osteophyte but remaining plantar to the dorsomedial cutaneous nerve. Blunt dissection down the bone is performed. Caution should be taken to avoid damaging the dorsomedial cutaneous nerve during this procedure due to its proximity to the portal.
3. A curved elevator is used to lift the capsule off the dorsal osteophyte proximally and dorsally to free up space for the burr.
4. A 3.1-mm wedge burr then is inserted and then advanced directly into the osteophyte running at low speed but high torque to minimize heat generation. Irrigation should be used to cool the burr, the bone, and the soft tissues. The surgeon should not try to approach the osteophyte dorsally because this endangers the extensor hallucis tendon and the medial sensory cutaneous nerve. Rather, the burr should engage the osteophyte from the base in a dorsal direction and advanced distally until the osteophyte is completely removed. Caution should be taken to avoid plantarflexing the hallux during this process because this may risk further injury to the extensor tendons.
5. The burr may be used to grind down the osteophyte, or a pituitary rongeur may be inserted to grasp and remove pieces of the osteophyte. A rasp can be used to remove large bone fragments or fragments adherent to the capsule. An angiocatheter may be used to irrigate the area completely.
6. Fluoroscopy may be used during resection to ensure that adequate bone has been removed and that all bone debris has been completely flushed out (**Fig. 24**). An opacity

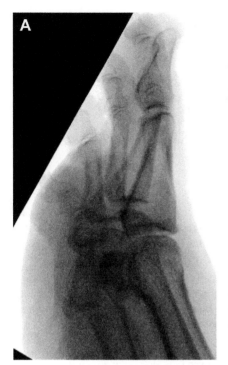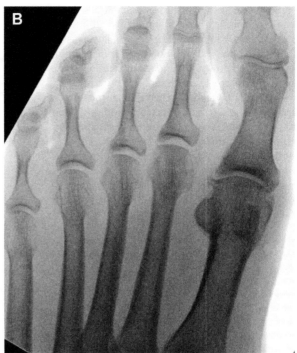

Fig. 24. (*A*, *B*) Final AP and lateral fluoroscopic views confirming complete resection of the dorsal osteophyte.

dorsal to the resection is indicative of likely remaining debris that requires further removal.

7. The amount of bone resected depends on surgeon preference.

8. If medial metatarsal osteophytes are present, these can be removed via the aforementioned technique through the same dorsomedial portal. If lateral metatarsal osteophytes are present, these can be removed via an additional incision dorsolaterally, adjacent to the initial incision.

9. The portals are closed with adhesive strips and simple dry dressing bandages.

Postoperative Care

- Patients immediately go into a stiff-soled shoe, with weight bearing as tolerated.
- The dry dressing may be removed at day 3, but the incision protected with a small bandage for 2 weeks.
- Simple range-of-motion exercises of the hallux can begin immediately after surgery.
- Patients may return to their own footwear on postoperative day 3 and may resume all tolerated activity after 2 weeks when the wound is healed.

Complications and Management

- Infection
  - Superficial infections may be treated with oral antibiotics, whereas deep infections may necessitate irrigation and débridement.
- Dorsomedial cutaneous nerve injury
  - This is an iatrogenic complication that has been cited to occur in 3% of cases.
  - Teoh and colleagues showed damage to the nerve in 15% of cases in a cadaveric study, highlighting the importance of adequate pocket space for the burr and making the nerve prior to incision whenever possible to mitigate risk.
- Persistent pain and worsening arthritis
  - This may necessitate either repeat cheilectomy and/or progression to fusion of the joint.

MINIMALLY INVASIVE FIRST METATARSOPHALANGEAL JOINT ARTHRODESIS

Introduction and Background for Minimally Invasive First Metatarsophalangeal Joint Arthrodesis

Hallux rigidus is a common cause of first MTPJ pain and stiffness. Fusion of the first MTPJ has a high union rate, and open techniques have been the historical gold standard for treatment of end-stage hallux rigidus. Minimally invasive techniques offer the potential for reduced pain, swelling, and lower wound complication rate. Limited literature exists describing outcomes after minimally invasive first MTPJ arthrodesis. A case series of 26 patients reported a fusion rate of 93%, very good patient satisfaction, and significant improvement in MOxFQ score.[22] Another series of 32 patients demonstrated a fusion rate of 97% with one deep infection using a percutaneous technique for first MTPJ arthrodesis.[23] There was a significant improvement in AOFAS score and high patient satisfaction.

Surgical Technique for Minimally Invasive First Metatarsophalangeal Joint Arthrodesis
Preoperative planning

- Consider patient bone quality and any prior hardware in place.

Indications

- Stages II–IV hallux rigidus that have failed conservative management.
- Stages II–IV hallux rigidus that have not responded to first MTPJ dorsal cheilectomy.

Contraindications

- Diffuse large osteophyte formation at the first MTPJ (relative).

Preparation and patient positioning

- The patient typically is positioned supine with the operative foot off of the bed distally and a bump under the hip on the operative side.
- The operative leg is elevated on a bump or blankets.
- The nonoperative leg may be frog-legged proximally away from the field and taped.
- The mini C-arm typically is positioned to the right of the patient for right-handed surgeons and to the left of the patient for left-handed surgeons, although this may be altered based on surgeon preference.

Minimally Invasive First Metatarsophalangeal Joint Arthrodesis

1. AP and lateral fluoroscopy views are used to place two .062 K-wires from dorsal to plantar 2 mm from the base of the hallux proximal phalanx joint surface (**Fig. 25**).

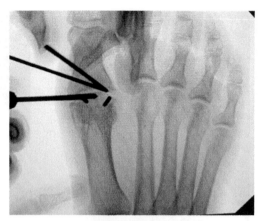

Fig. 25. Intraoperative AP fluoroscopic view demonstrating proper k wire placement.

2. A midaxial 4-mm medial portal at the level of the first MTPJ then is created using a #15 blade with use of AP fluoroscopy views.
3. A straight hemostat is used to bluntly dissect into the first MTPJ.
4. The 3-mm wedge burr is inserted into the first MTPJ via the medial portal.
5. The 3.1-mm wedge burr is used to resect the first MTPJ surface with AP fluoroscopic guidance along the K-wires to limit bone loss during joint preparation (**Fig. 26**).
   a. Be sure to irrigate the burr during use to prevent skin thermal injury.
6. A dorsal longitudinal first MTPJ incision and capsulotomy are made to evaluate joint preparation.
   a. There usually is some remaining cartilage at the apex of the concavity of the hallux base of the proximal phalanx.
7. A small curved curette is used to remove any remaining first MTPJ cartilage.
8. The joint is irrigated with normal saline.

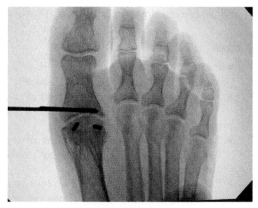

Fig. 26. Intraoperative AP fluoroscopic view demonstrating burr insertion via the medial portal.

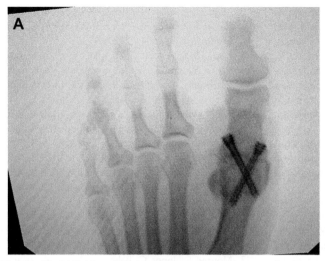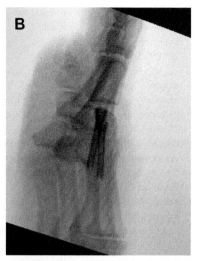

Fig. 27. Final (A) AP and (B) lateral fluoroscopic views confirming screw placement and fusion of the first MTPJ.

9. A K-wire or small drill is used to fenestrate both sides of the joint.
10. The joint is irrigated fully. Bone graft may be placed in the joint to facilitate fusion healing per surgeon preference. The joint then is compressed, reduced, and held with 2 to 3 crossing wires. Fluoroscopy confirms compression across the joint, reduction of any deformity, and satisfactory positioning of the wires.
11. The wires then are measured and overdrilled, and then 2 to 3 cannulated screws are placed, with compression delivered alternately on each screw. AP and lateral fluoroscopic views confirm proper placement (Fig. 27).
12. The portals are closed with sutures or adhesive strips and simple dry dressing bandages are applied.

Postoperative Care

- The patient is placed in a flat postoperative shoe or heel-wedge front off-loading shoe and allowed weight bearing as tolerated.
- The dressing is removed at 2 weeks postoperatively.
- Six weeks to 10 weeks postoperatively, depending on the degree of bone healing, the patient may transition to a supportive footwear with a rocker bottom sole.

Complications and Management

- Infection

  - Irrigation and débridement are recommended for deep infections.
- Nonunion
  - Full radiographic bony union across the osteotomy may take 3 months to 6 months. In patients with persistent pain, a nonunion may be present. CT scan may be considered. Revision with compression plate and/or screws is recommended when present.
- Skin thermal burn
  - Recommend avoidance of tourniquet and irrigation of the burr to prevent thermal injury.

ACKNOWLEDGMENTS

Dr A.H. Johnson would like to profusely thank Drs David Redfern and Joel Vernois for introducing her to percutaneous surgery and for their continued teaching and mentorship.

DISCLOSURE

O.N. Schipper: DePuy, a Johnson & Johnson Company: paid consultant; Medline: paid consultant; and Novastep: IP royalties and paid consultant. J. Day: nothing to disclose. G.S. Ray: nothing to disclose. A.H. Johnson: American Orthopaedic Foot and Ankle Society: board or committee member; AOFAMIS: board or committee member; Medartis: paid consultant; Novastep: IP royalties; paid consultant; and Synthes: paid consultant.

REFERENCES

1. Vernois J, Redfern D, Ferraz L, et al. Minimally invasive surgery osteotomy of the hindfoot. Clin Podiatr Med Surg 2015;32(3):419–34.

2. Redfern D, Gill I, Harris M. Early experience with a minimally invasive modified chevron and akin osteotomy for correction of hallux valgus. 2011;93(SUPP_IV):482.

3. Lai MC, Rikhraj IS, Woo YL, et al. Clinical and radiological outcomes comparing percutaneous chevron-akin osteotomies vs open scarf-akin osteotomies for hallux valgus. Foot Ankle Int 2018;39(3):311–7.

4. Lee M, Walsh J, Smith MM, et al. Hallux valgus correction comparing percutaneous chevron/Akin (PECA) and open scarf/Akin osteotomies. Foot Ankle Int 2017;38(8):838–46.

5. Kendal AR, Khalid A, Ball T, et al. Complications of minimally invasive calcaneal osteotomy versus open osteotomy. Foot Ankle Int 2015;36(6):685–90.

6. Stiglitz Y, Cazeau C. Minimally invasive surgery and percutaneous surgery of the hindfoot and midfoot. Eur J Orthop Surg Traumatol 2018;28(5):839–47.

7. Gutteck N, Zeh A, Wohlrab D, et al. Comparative results of percutaneous calcaneal osteotomy in correction of hindfoot deformities. Foot Ankle Int 2019;40(3):276–81.

8. DiDomenico LA, Anain J, Wargo-Dorsey M. Assessment of medial and lateral neurovascular structures after percutaneous posterior calcaneal displacement osteotomy: a cadaver study. J Foot Ankle Surg 2011;50(6):668–71.

9. Tennant JN, Veljkovic A, Phisitkul P. Technique tip: percutaneous endoscopically-assisted calcaneal slide osteotomy. Iowa Orthop J 2013;33:191–5.

10. Abbasian A, Zaidi R, Guha A, et al. Comparison of three different fixation methods of calcaneal osteotomies. Foot Ankle Int 2013;34(3):420–5.

11. Highlander P, VonHerbulis E, Gonzalez A, et al. Complications of the weil osteotomy. Foot Ankle Spec 2011;4(3):165–70.

12. Migues A, Slullitel G, Bilbao F, et al. Floating-toe deformity as a complication of the weil osteotomy. Foot Ankle Int 2004;25(9):609–13.

13. Haque S, Kakwani R, Chadwick C, et al. Outcome of minimally invasive distal metatarsal metaphyseal osteotomy (DMMO) for lesser toe metatarsalgia. Foot Ankle Int 2016;37(1):58–63.

14. Teoh KH, Hariharan K. Minimally invasive distal metatarsal metaphyseal osteotomy (DMMO) of the fifth metatarsal for bunionette correction. Foot Ankle Int 2018;39(4):450–7.

15. Walter R, Perera A. Open, arthroscopic, and percutaneous cheilectomy for hallux rigidus. Foot Ankle Clin 2015;20(3):421–31.

16. Teoh KH, Tan WT, Atiyah Z, et al. Clinical outcomes following minimally invasive dorsal cheilectomy for hallux rigidus. Foot Ankle Int 2019;40(2):195–201.

17. Morgan S, Jones C, Palmer S. Minimally invasive cheilectomy: Functional outcome and comparison with open cheilectomy. 2012;94(SUPP_XLIII):14.

18. Dawe E, Ball T, Annamalai S, et al. Early results of minimally invasive cheilectomy for painful hallux rigidus. 2012;94(SUPP_XXII):33.

19. Loveday D, Guha A, Singh D. Arthritis great toe MTPJ. Consensus of the round table. Aspects of orthopaedic foot and ankle surgery. Paris. 2012:1–9.

20. Razik A, Sott A. Cheilectomy for hallux rigidus. Foot Ankle Clin 2016;21(3):451–7.

21. Redfern D, Vernois J, Legré BP. Percutaneous surgery of the forefoot. Clin Podiatr Med Surg 2015; 32(3):291–332.

22. Fanous RN, Ridgers S, Sott AH. Minimally invasive arthrodesis of the first metatarsophalangeal joint for hallux rigidus. Foot Ankle Surg 2014;20(3):170–3.

23. Bauer T, Lortat-Jacob A, Hardy P. First metatarsophalangeal joint percutaneous arthrodesis. Orthop Traumatol Surg Res 2010;96(5):567–73.

Special Article

Deep Venous Thrombosis and Pulmonary Embolism After Minimally Invasive Transforaminal Lumbar Interbody Fusion

Report of 2 Cases in 315 Procedures

Catherine R. Olinger, MD*, Raymond J. Gardocki, MD

KEYWORDS

- Minimally invasive spine surgery • Transforaminal lumbar interbody fusion • Pulmonary embolism
- Deep venous thrombosis

KEY POINTS

- Deep venous thrombosis (DVT) and pulmonary embolism (PE) are uncommon in patients with minimally invasive transforaminal lumbar interbody fusion.
- Following the guidelines of the North American Spine Society concerning DVT prophylaxis resulted in only 2 instances of DVT and PE in 315 procedures.
- Older age and obesity tend to be risk factors for the development of DVT and PE.
- Mechanical DVT prophylaxis appears to be adequate in patients undergoing elective spinal surgery.

For nearly 3 decades, transforaminal lumbar interbody fusion (TLIF) has been a widely used procedure for the treatment of degenerative lumbar disorders, providing circumferential spinal fusion, restoration of disk height, and maintenance of normal lumbar lordosis. Despite high fusion rates (95%), TLIF requires extensive paravertebral muscle stripping and retraction, damaging the paraspinous muscles and nerves.[1,2] Advances in imaging and instrumentation have led to the development of minimally invasive transforaminal lumbar interbody fusion (MITLIF) techniques.[3–5] Both techniques have low complication rates, and deep venous thrombosis (DVT) and pulmonary embolism (PE) are especially uncommon, reported to occur in from fewer than 0.5% to 4.0% of patients in most studies. Although exceedingly rare, DVT

and PE can have serious consequences, including cardiopulmonary instability and death. We report 2 patients with MITLIF procedures who developed DVT/PE.

In a series of 315 patients with MITLIF procedures, only 2 (0.6%) developed DVT/PE. All patients were treated immediately after surgery with thromboembolism-deterrent (TED) hose and mechanical DVT prophylaxis with calf sequential compression devices (SCDs). No pharmacologic DVT prophylaxis was given. This postoperative management protocol was based on the North American Spine Society (NASS) guidelines.[6]

CASE REPORTS

Case 1

A 72-year-old morbidly obese man presented with a 4-year history of buttock and leg pain

---

Department of Orthopaedic Surgery and Biomedical Engineering, University of Tennessee-Campbell Clinic, 1211 Union Avenue, Suite 510, Memphis, TN 38104, USA
* Corresponding author.
E-mail address: colinger@campbellclinic.com

Orthop Clin N Am 51 (2020) 423–425
https://doi.org/10.1016/j.ocl.2020.02.006
0030-5898/20/© 2020 Elsevier Inc. All rights reserved.

that had become worse over the past year. He was able to walk only 60 feet before progressive leg pain and weakness became so severe that he could not walk farther. Comorbidities included hypertension (HTN) and obstructive sleep apnea (OSA). Several epidural injections had provided temporary relief, but the pain and weakness persisted. Electromyography (EMG) and nerve conduction studies showed polyradiculopathy consistent with multilevel stenosis. MRI demonstrated multilevel lumbar foraminal stenosis and canal stenosis.

He was treated with multilevel MITLIF from L2 to S1 with pedicle screw fixation and bone morphogenetic protein. The operative time was 5 hours. TED hose and mechanical DVT prophylaxis with calf SCDs bilaterally were used immediately after surgery. No pharmacologic DVT prophylaxis was given. There were no immediate postoperative complications, and the patient was independently ambulatory on the day of surgery. He was discharged to home 2 days after surgery.

Six days after surgery, the patient presented to the emergency room complaining of confusion and difficulty breathing. Examination found right lower extremity DVT with a saddle PE. He was treated with thrombolysis, inferior vena cava (IVC) filter placement, and intubation for respiratory failure. When he recovered from the embolism, he was placed on long-term anticoagulation medication. His spine fusion healed, with resolution of leg pain and weakness. At 4-year follow-up, he had experienced no further complications.

Case 2

A 69-year-old obese man presented with a 9-year history of leg pain and weakness that had progressively worsened. He described an aching pain that radiated to his left buttock and lateral ankle in the L5 distribution; pain was not relieved with medication, and an L5 discectomy 9 years earlier had failed to resolve his pain. Comorbidities included HTN, OSA, diabetes mellitus, and coronary artery disease. MRI demonstrated spondylolisthesis at the L4-5 level with a large central herniation into a severely stenotic canal.

He was treated with multilevel MITLIF from L4 to L5 with pedicle screw fixation and bone morphogenetic protein. The operative time was 3 hours and 28 minutes. TED hose and mechanical DVT prophylaxis with calf SCDs bilaterally were used immediately after surgery. No pharmacologic DVT prophylaxis was given. There were no immediate postoperative complications, and the patient was independently

ambulatory on the day of surgery. He was discharged to home 2 days after surgery. Five days after surgery the patient presented complaining of constant right leg pain. He was found to have right lower extremity DVT and a PE that required placement of an IVC filter and anticoagulation medication. His fusion healed uneventfully, and his leg pain and weakness resolved. At 2-year follow-up, he had experienced no further complications.

DISCUSSION

Vascular complications such as DVT and PE are rare after both standard TLIF and MITLIF. Reports in the literature describe occurrence rates ranging from 0.4% to 4.0%,[7–11] with at least 1 large study (300 patients) reporting no DVT or PE.[12] In their systematic review and meta-analysis, Bernatz and Anderson[13] found only 2 of 13 studies reporting DVT/PE as the cause of 30-day readmissions. Although uncommon, DVT/PE can have devastating consequences. Wong and colleagues[11] reported 1 death secondary to a massive PE in 513 patients with MITLIF; another 6 patients had either DVT or PE that required anticoagulation therapy. The frequency of these complications in our 315 patients (0.6%) is similar to that reported by others.

Although DVT/PE has not been shown to be more frequent after MITLIF than after standard TLIF, some have postulated that the longer operative time generally required for MITLIF may be a contributing factor.[7] The operative times (5 hours and 3 hours and 28 minutes) in our 2 patients with DVT/PE were somewhat longer than the usual operative time for standard MITLIF, but not significantly so. MITLIF has a definite learning curve, and as our experience has increased to more than 100 cases, operative times have decreased, and no DVT/PE complications have occurred over the past 6 years with the use of calf SCDs.

Both patients with DVT/PE were elderly obese men with multiple comorbidities, and both were treated with mechanical DVT prophylaxis, as outlined in the guidelines, which do not support routine chemical prophylaxis for patients with elective spine procedures. Some studies have suggested age and obesity as factors contributing to more frequent complications after spine surgery, whereas others have found no differences between outcomes in obese and nonobese patients[14–18] or in older patients.[9] We believe this infrequent occurrence of DVT/PE (0.6%) supports the continued use of the NASS guidelines in patients undergoing MITLIF.

DISCLOSURE

Dr R.J. Gardocki is a speaker for JoiMax; Dr C.R. Olinger has nothing to disclose.

REFERENCES

1. Fan S, Hu Z, Zhao F, et al. Multifidus muscle changes and clinical effects of one-level posterior lumbar interbody fusion: minimally invasive procedure versus conventional open approach. Eur Spine J 2010;19(2):316–24.
2. Kawaguchi Y, Matsui H, Tsuji H. Back muscle injury after posterior lumbar spine surgery. Part 2: histologic and histochemical analyses in humans. Spine (Phila Pa 1976) 1994;19:2598–602.
3. Perez-Cruet MJ, Hussain N, White GZ, et al. Quality-of-life outcomes with minimally invasive transforaminal lumbar interbody fusion based on long-term analysis of 304 consecutive patients. Spine (Phila Pa 1976) 2014;39(3):E191–8.
4. Schwender J, Holly L, Rouben D, et al. Minimally invasive transforaminal lumbar interbody fusion (TLIF): technical feasibility and initial results. J Spinal Disord Tech 2005;18(Suppl):S1–6.
5. Shunwu F, Xing Z, Fengdong Z, et al. Minimally invasive transforaminal lumbar interbody fusion for the treatment of degenerative lumbar diseases. Spine (Phila Pa 1976) 2010;35(17):1615–20.
6. North American Spine Society Clinical Guidelines for Multidisciplinary Spine Care. Antithrombotic Therapies in Spine Surgery. Burr Ridge (IL). 2009. Available at: https://www.spine.org/Research-Clinical-Care/Quality-Improvement/Clinical-Guidelines. Accessed January 13, 2020.
7. Hey HW, Hee HT. Open and minimally invasive transforaminal lumbar interbody fusion: comparison of intermediate results and complications. Asian Spine J 2015;9(2):185–93.
8. Hu W, Tang J, Wu X, et al. Minimally invasive versus open transforaminal lumbar fusion: a systematic review of complications. Int Orthop 2016;40(9):1883–90.
9. Lin GX, Quillo-Olvera J, Jo HJ, et al. Minimally invasive transforaminal lumbar interbody fusion: a comparison study based on endplate subsidence and cystic change in individuals above and below the age of 65. World Neurosurg 2017;106:174–84.
10. Tsahtsarlis A, Wood M. Minimally invasive transforaminal lumbar interbody fusion and degenerative lumbar spine disease. Eur Spine J 2012;21(11):2300–5.
11. Wong AP, Smith ZA, Nixon AT, et al. Intraoperative and perioperative complications in minimally invasive transforaminal lumbar interbody fusion: a review of 513 patients. J Neurosurg Spine 2015;22(5):487–95.
12. Hari A, Krishna M, Rajagandhi S, et al. Minimally invasive transforaminal lumbar interbody fusion—indications and clinical experience. Neurol India 2016;64(3):444–54.
13. Bernatz JT, Anderson PA. Thirty-day readmission rates in spine surgery: systematic review and meta-analysis. Neurosurg Focus 2015;39(4):E7.
14. Buerba RA, Fu MC, Gruskay JA, et al. Obese Class III patients at significantly greater risk of multiple complications after lumbar surgery: an analysis of 10,387 patients in the ACS NSQIP database. Spine J 2014;14(9):2008–18.
15. Lau D, Ziewacz J, Park P. Minimally invasive transforaminal lumbar interbody fusion for spondylolisthesis in patients with significant obesity. J Clin Neurosci 2013;20(1):80–3.
16. Park P, Upadhyaya C, Garton HJ, et al. The impact of minimally invasive spine surgery on perioperative complications in overweight or obese patients. Neurosurgery 2008;62(3):693–9.
17. Senker W, Meznik C, Avian A, et al. Perioperative morbidity and complications in minimal access surgery techniques in obese patients with degenerative lumbar disease. Eur Spine J 2011;20(7):1182–7.
18. Wang YP, An JL, Sun YP, et al. Comparison of outcomes between minimally invasive transforaminal lumbar interbody fusion and traditional posterior lumbar intervertebral fusion in obese patients with lumbar disk prolapse. Ther Clin Risk Manag 2017;13:87–94.

Printed and bound by CPI Group (UK) Ltd, Croydon, CR0 4YY

03/10/2024

01040371-0012